Health Systems
Science Review

Health Systems Science Review

Jesse M. Ehrenfeld, MD, MPH, FAMIA, FASA

Joseph A. Johnson, Jr., Distinguished Leadership Professor
Professor of Anesthesiology, Surgery, Biomedical Informatics &
   Health Policy
Director, Education Research – Office of Health Sciences
   Education
Director, Program for LGBTQ Health
Associate Director, Vanderbilt Anesthesiology & Perioperative
   Informatics Research Division
Vanderbilt University School of Medicine
Nashville, TN

Jed D. Gonzalo, MD, MSc

Associate Dean, Health Systems Education, College of Medicine
   (Hershey)
Associate Professor, Department of Medicine
Associate Professor, Department of Public Health Sciences
Penn State College of Medicine
Hershey, PA

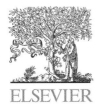

ELSEVIER

HEALTH SYSTEMS SCIENCE REVIEW   ISBN: 978-0-323-65370-1

Library of Congress Control Number: 2019934395

Content Strategist: Elyse O'Grady
Content Development Specialist: Caroline Dorey-Stein
Publishing Services Manager: Catherine Jackson
Project Manager: Tara Delaney
Design Direction: Margaret Reid

Printed in Canada.
Last digit is the print number: 9   8   7   6   5   4   3   2   1

ELSEVIER

1600 John F. Kennedy Blvd.
Ste 1600
Philadelphia, PA 19103-2899

Foreword

Mastery of health systems science provides a fundamental understanding of how health care is delivered, how health care professionals work together to deliver that care, and how the health system can improve patient care. It includes content in health care delivery and processes, health care policy and economics, clinical informatics, social determinants of health, population and public health, patient safety, quality improvement, value in health care, teamwork and collaboration, leadership, and systems thinking. Health systems science has been called the third pillar of health professions education—a required addition to the historic disciplines of basic and clinical sciences.

The editors and authors of this review textbook have extensive experience in teaching health systems science in a broad variety of settings and are the leading experts from the AMA Accelerating Change in Medical Education Consortium schools. The book includes 11 chapters on key health systems science topics. Each chapter includes numerous cases and approximately 25 multiple choice questions. Answers are fully explained at the end of the chapter.

This review book is meant to prepare medical and health professions students to be assessed in their understanding of health systems science and its core subjects. It can provide valuable self-assessment and topic mastery guidance for anyone wishing to improve their learning and expertise in these important domains.

Susan E. Skochelak, MD, MPH
Group Vice President, Medical Education
American Medical Association

Preface

Health care delivery in the United States is rapidly evolving to better achieve the desired outcomes of patients' experience of care, population health, decreasing costs, and improved clinician wellness. These shifts have stimulated an aggressive reframing of medical education to better align with these needs, notably by better preparing learners to be better prepared to practice and lead in complex health care settings and meet the needs of patients. Since 2013, the American Medical Association (AMA) has cultivated a learning community to accelerate changes in medical education to help contribute to and meet the needs of learners and patients. Complementing the traditional basic and clinical sciences, the third pillar of medical education—Health Systems Science—was developed as the comprehensive framework that pulls together the breadth of systems-based competencies that allow learners and clinicians to function and optimize health care outcomes. The Health Systems Science pillar includes concepts and competencies related to health care policy and economics, public and population health, social determinants of health, interprofessional collaboration, clinical informatics, value-based care (including patient safety), health system improvement, and systems thinking. Each of these individual concept areas existed before in education, but they operated in a disconnected manner and with limited penetration into core curricula. The Health Systems Science comprehensive framework provides the cohesive and integrated structure into which core educational programs and learners' knowledge and skills can be best operationalized. In short, the Health Systems Science framework is facilitating a new era of medical education reform.

Complementing the core Health Systems Science textbook, this Health Systems Science Review book is the first to unify the varied conceptual areas into one knowledge-based resource across all of these critical areas. We hope this textbook will serve as a foundational resource for advancing the knowledge-based components of Health Systems Science for both learners and current-day clinicians.

The editors would like to thank the members of the AMA Accelerating Change in Medical Education Consortium for their dedication to advancing this field and their contributions to this work. We would like to dedicate this textbook to the patients, communities, and populations we serve, and the individuals who are actively embracing the much needed shifts in education and care delivery to meet the needs of our patients and health systems.

Jesse M. Ehrenfeld, MD, MPH
Jed D. Gonzalo, MD, MSc

Acknowledgements

The editors would like to thank the authors for all their hard work on their chapters, the American Medical Association (AMA) for supporting this project, and Victoria Stagg Elliott, technical writer for the AMA, for all her efforts to keep this project moving.

Contents

Health Systems
Science Review

Health Care Delivery and Process

Apoorve Nayyar, MBBS, Ugwuji Maduekwe, MD, MMSc

Cases and questions

Case 1

A hospital is undergoing consideration for a status change from a Level III trauma center (a center with resources available for emergency resuscitation, surgery, and intensive care of *most* trauma patients) to a Level II trauma center (a center with comprehensive multidisciplinary trauma care with all essential specialties available, but no teaching/research facilities). In addition to previously available services, it has added 24/7 coverage by specialties such as orthopedic surgery, neurosurgery, anesthesiology, emergency medicine, radiology, and critical care over the last 5 years. The hospital also implemented a quality assessment program to monitor performance metrics, including the duration of stay in the emergency department prior to definitive treatment, in-hospital length of stay, complications, unplanned 30-day readmissions, and overall mortality. With the hospital-wide transition to electronic health records and digital data entry, the center has been able to reduce the average wait time in the emergency department from 85 minutes to 45 minutes, 30-day readmission rate from 8.9% to 5.4%, and the overall mortality rate from 6.6% to 4.3%.

Q 1.1: Which of the following best describes the framework for improvements in health care delivery in this question?
a. Industrial quality management model
b. Donabedian model for care quality
c. Quality assurance model
d. Pay-for-performance (P4P) model

Case 2

Multiple studies have demonstrated that distance to care is the largest barrier for patients obtaining medical care for cardiac emergencies in Dallas County (Texas). Current lengthy distance to care leads to increased travel times and out-of-pocket health care costs, and less optimal cardiac outcomes in this patient population. A large hospital's cardiac care department is setting up five satellite clinics, located strategically throughout the county, to provide emergency and preventive services. Each practicing specialist physician of the department will see patients 1 day per week at these new clinics. This endeavor is also expected to lower the health care costs borne by the patient.

Q 2.1: From a public health perspective, which of the following best describes the primary goal of this new endeavor?
a. Increased patient referrals to the hospital
b. Increased patient outreach by the hospital
c. Improvement of the health of the population
d. Improvement in cardiac medical education

Q 2.2: Which of the following are defining characteristics of the Triple Aim of health care?
a. Improved health of the population, reduced health care costs, enhanced patient experience
b. Performance-based physician reimbursement, continuous quality improvement, prevention of physician burnout
c. Increased funding for health care research, reduced health care costs, performance-based reimbursement
d. Improvements in medical education, development of accountable care organizations, prevention of physician burnout

Q 2.3: Which of the following may be associated with the increased emphasis on the pursuit of the Triple Aim of health care?
a. Increased likelihood of medical errors
b. Compromised patient safety
c. Risk of health care worker burnout
d. Increased paperwork

Case 3

A 66-year-old female is brought to the emergency department an hour after an episode of loss of consciousness. The patient is accompanied by her adult daughter. The daughter states that the patient visited her primary care physician (PCP) this morning after a recent increase in thirst, water intake, and frequency of urination for the last week. The patient has a history of long-standing type 2 diabetes mellitus controlled with oral hypoglycemic agents combined with daily insulin. Upon blood analysis at the PCP's office, the patient's hemoglobin A1c (HbA1c) was found to be 9.1% with a blood glucose level of 321 mg/dL. The physician recommended a dosage adjustment for her daily insulin and ordered an immediate dose of "100u of regular human insulin." The nurse at the PCP's office administered the insulin, and the patient was brought home. However, 30 minutes after reaching home, the patient started feeling dizzy, sweating, and having palpitations. Soon after, the patient lost consciousness. The patient's daughter immediately administered oral glucose gel to the patient's buccal mucosa. Thereafter the patient regained consciousness and was brought to the emergency department. Upon review of the insulin dosage, it was found out that the nurse misread the "100**u** of regular human insulin" as "100**0** of regular human insulin" and administered 1000 units of insulin.

Q 3.1: Which of the following is most likely to have prevented this medication error?
a. Direct verbal communication from the physician to the nurse
b. Computerized prescription entry and medication dispensing
c. Administration of the medication (and appropriate dose) by the physician
d. Decentralized pharmacy system

Case 4

A 27-year-old nurse works on the in-patient floor unit of vascular surgery with 20 beds arranged in a rectangular layout. He works 10-hour shifts every day and is usually in charge of the care of four to five patients. This vascular surgery unit is located next to a busy hallway that connects two buildings of the hospital. The supply closet for the unit is in the far end of the unit and the nurses' workstation is at the opposite end of the unit.

Q 4.1: Which of the following changes to the design of the unit is most likely to improve the efficiency of the health care providers working in this unit?
a. Radial layout of the beds
b. Central location of the supplies closet
c. Central location of the nurses' workstation
d. All of the above

Q 4.2: The nurses working in this unit have, on average, higher stress and anxiety scores compared to other surgical floor units' nurses with a similar patient workload. Which of the following design modifications would be the most effective means to reduce the stress level and increase the efficiency of the health care providers in this unit?
a. Location of the unit closer to the elevator
b. Increased lighting
c. Availability of healthy behavioral options (e.g., healthy food choices)
d. Reduction in the noise level

Case 5

A 36-year-old plastic surgeon has just joined a new health care organization as a practicing physician. Per her contract, the physician is expected to dedicate 80% of her time to clinical services and 20% to research. However, due to the current paucity of plastic surgeons in the organization, she is constantly overbooked for procedures and ends up spending nearly all of her time engaged in clinical activities, leaving little or no time for research during the week. She works on her research projects over the weekends.

Q 5.1: Which of the following would have been affected the most if the physician had not been able to adjust the extra clinical workload in her schedule?
a. Patient–physician interaction
b. Operational capacity of the organization
c. Operational effectiveness of the organization
d. Quality of patient care
e. Health care costs of plastic surgery procedures

Q 5.2: If this pattern of work overload persists continuously, which of the following may have the most significant impact on patient care?
a. Increased physician stress
b. Increased patient wait time
c. Medical errors
d. Increasing health care costs to patient
e. Reduced patient–physician interaction

Case 6

At her quarterly performance evaluation meeting with her boss, the physician is told to "pick up the slack," "adjust to things the way they are," and that her clinical results "aren't that great" despite excellent patient-reported outcomes. Her request for more personnel or physician partners' support to balance the clinical workload is not met. This continues for 3 years at which point the physician feels fatigue that does not respond to adequate rest. She feels emotionally exhausted and helpless and is increasingly cynical. She no longer feels the motivation to go to work and feels that her work constantly lacks meaning.

Q 6.1: What is this physician currently experiencing?
a. Adjustment disorder
b. Physician exhaustion
c. Physician burnout
d. Major depressive disorder

Q 6.2: Which of the following measures by the physician could have potentially prevented burnout in this physician?
a. Regular physical exercise
b. Mindfulness-based meditation
c. Stress management strategies
d. Spending time on hobbies
e. All of the above
f. None of the above

Q 6.3: Which of the following measures by the health care organization could have potentially prevented burnout in this physician?
a. Provision of regular counseling services
b. Better ergonomic design of the workplace
c. Better resource allocation
d. Better environmental design of the facility

Case 7

A previously healthy 59-year-old woman presents to the surgical oncology clinic after an abnormal mammogram revealed a round, smooth mass in the left breast as well as an irregular mass in the right breast. After bilateral stereotactic biopsies, the mass on the left is determined to be a fibroadenoma and the irregular mass in the right breast is established to be invasive ductal carcinoma of the breast. She elects to undergo lumpectomy with sentinel lymph node biopsy on the right breast with a plan for postoperative radiation therapy. On the day of the planned surgery, the patient is greeted by the surgical resident assigned to the case who discusses the procedure with the patient and obtains the patient's consent for the surgery in the preoperative care area. The patient is taken to the operative room (OR) and undergoes surgery on the left side. The mass excised is confirmed to be a fibroadenoma.

Q 7.1: Which of the following best describes this situation?
a. Never event
b. Near miss event
c. Adverse event
d. Malpractice

Q 7.2: Which of the following may have prevented this from happening?
a. Surgical site marking
b. Timeout before the start of the procedure
c. Attending surgeon meeting and discussing the procedure with the patient in preoperative care
d. Coordination between the preoperative care staff and the OR team
e. Review of patient's disease history by the OR staff
f. All of the above

Q 7.3: Subsequently, the patient undergoes breast conserving surgery on the right side and the malignant tumor is removed. Who would bear the health care cost of the additional surgery?
a. Patient
b. Health insurance payer
c. Centers for Medicare and Medicaid Services (CMS)
d. Hospital

Q 7.4: Which of the following may also be classified as a "never event"?
a. Nosocomial infections
b. Wrong-site procedure
c. Sacral (decubitus) ulcers
d. In-hospital fall/trauma
e. All of the above

Case 8

A 76-year-old African American male presents to the clinic with increased fatigue over the last 6 months. He has noted a change in bowel and the presence of bright red blood in stool.

The fecal occult blood testing is found to be positive and upon colonoscopy, a mass was identified in the left colon. A diagnosis of adenocarcinoma of the colon is confirmed, and the patient is scheduled for a hemicolectomy. Due to his age and infirmities, he is admitted preoperatively. The patient is assisted with a bowel preparation and chlorhexidine wash by the nursing staff on the surgical unit. On the day of surgery, he is taken to the OR. There, the team of surgeons, anesthesiologists, nurses, and technicians coordinate to perform the hemicolectomy. Upon completion of the procedure, the anesthesia is reversed, and the patient is transferred to the postoperative care team. The postoperative care team monitors the patient's vital signs postoperatively until the patient is ready to be returned to the surgical floor.

Q 8.1: In the milieu of health care structures, what does each unit of clinical teams (e.g., preoperative staff, OR team, postoperative care team) represent?
a. Microsystem
b. Mesosystem
c. Macrosystem
d. Health care ecosystem

Case 9

Two years after initial treatment, the patient suffers a thromboembolic event affecting the right middle cerebral artery. After initial stabilization in the hospital, the patient is determined to have a residual left deficit affecting his speech, gait, and motor function. He is unable to perform independently the activities of daily living.

Q 9.1: After discharge from the hospital, which of the following facilities would be ideal for this patient's recovery?
a. Hospice care facility
b. Ambulatory care center
c. Specialty hospital
d. Skilled nursing facility
e. Outpatient care

Case 10

A 61-year-old Caucasian male presents to the emergency department with chest pain of an hour's duration. The patient was engaging in sexual activity when the pain started. It is crushing, substernal, persistent, and radiating toward his left shoulder. The pain does not vary with a change in position. The patient has a past medical history of diabetes mellitus, hypertension, hyperlipidemia, and chronic stable angina. He is afebrile (98.7°F), has a heart rate of 116 beats per minutes (bpm), and blood pressure 118/88 mmHg. His current electrocardiogram (ECG) demonstrates ST segment elevation and large peaked T waves. The blood work shows elevation in creatine phosphokinase MB (CK-MB) and troponins. The patient is immediately given sublingual nitroglycerin, provided with continuous oxygen administration, given a dose of aspirin with clopidogrel, and placed on cardiac monitoring. Shortly after, the patient's blood pressure drops to 80/50 mmHg and his chest pain worsens. Upon further investigation, it is discovered that the patient had consumed a 50-mg tablet of sildenafil prior to engaging in sexual activity.

Q 10.1: Which of the following is the most likely cause of the patient's current condition?
a. Prescription error
b. Adverse drug reaction
c. Drug interaction
d. Anaphylactic reaction

Q 10.2: Which of the following may have prevented such an event from occurring?
a. Assessment of blood nitrate levels
b. Urine toxicology screen
c. Medication reconciliation at admission
d. Lower dose of nitroglycerin

Case 10, continued

The patient is stabilized and receives percutaneous coronary angiography that demonstrates a 95% occlusion of the left anterior descending artery. He undergoes coronary artery bypass grafting with an uneventful postoperative period. Twelve days later the patient is being discharged to home.

Q 10.3: Which of the following would be most helpful at this time to prevent any further medication errors?
a. Calling the patient's primary care physician to discuss hospital course
b. Appropriate documentation of patient's hospital course
c. Giving the patient a copy of the medical records
d. Explaining the hospital course to the patient and asking him to convey it to the primary care physician

Case 11

A 66-year-old Caucasian female with longstanding left knee osteoarthritis presents to an orthopedic surgeon's office for a surgical management consult. The patient has been using acetaminophen and oral nonsteroidal antiinflammatory drugs for the past 20 years for pain relief. In the past 3 years, the patient has also received intraarticular corticosteroid injections. She states that the pain is unbearable and inquires about prosthetic knee replacement. A decision to undergo knee arthroplasty is made, and subsequently the patient undergoes the procedure with minor complications. The hospital's charges for the procedure total $21,184, but her insurance company gives the hospital $15,384, in line with a previously agreed upon amount allocated for all surgical care related to knee osteoarthritis.

Q 11.1: Which payment model does this scenario best represent?
a. Shared savings/one-sided risk model
b. Patient-centered medical home (PCMH)
c. Provider-sponsored health plan (PSHP)
d. Capitation model
e. Bundled payment model

Q 11.2: How could the reimbursement change if the patient was on a traditional fee-for-service model?
a. Increase
b. Decrease
c. No change
d. Paid by the patient

Q 11.3: What parameter of health care delivery is NOT accounted for in the traditional fee-for-service model, as opposed to the value-based model?
a. Volume of patients treated
b. Total number of services provided per patient
c. Cost of the health care
d. Quality of the health care

Case 12

A 67-year-old male with a longstanding history of diabetes mellitus recently developed an ulcer on the plantar surface of the right foot. Despite adequate wound care and antibiotic coverage, the wound has not healed completely. The patient's PCP refers the patient to the nearby hospital's foot clinic. This hospital recently partnered with this PCP and several other physicians operating independently in the nearby area to provide comprehensive care to the community. The patient is seen by a vascular surgeon and a podiatrist. The patient is provided a pressure offloading device for the foot, in addition to wound care and antibiotic agents. An endocrinologist is also consulted to manage the patient's blood glucose levels. The patient's wound heals in 2 weeks. This combined team of physicians is reimbursed by the payer upon evaluation of the patient's clinical management plan, quality of care, and overall cost to the organization. Upon follow-up with the PCP, the PCP emphasizes the need for modifications to diet and regular exercise, in addition to compliance with the medication regimen.

Q 12.1: Which of the following does this consortium of health care providers represent?
a. Group practice
b. Accountable care organization
c. Health management organization
d. Patient-centered medical home

Case 13

A 49-year-old Caucasian female presents to the clinic with 8 days of colicky right upper quadrant pain. The pain typically occurs after meals, lasts for 1 to 2 hours, and is associated with nausea and vomiting. Since yesterday, the pain has become severe and is now constant. The patient's current pulse is 114/min, respirations 18/min, and temperature 38.4°C (101.2°F). The patient's height is 61 inches (156 cm), weight 223 lb (101 kg), and BMI 42.1 kg/m². The patient has a past medical history of hypertension, hyperlipidemia, and chronic obstructive pulmonary disease (COPD). Upon examination, there is pain on palpation of the right upper quadrant and Murphy sign is elicited. Ultrasonography shows the presence of gallstones in the gallbladder. The patient undergoes laparoscopic cholecystectomy and is transferred to the surgical floor after 2 hours in the postoperative unit. On postoperative day 3, her temperature is 39.1°C (102.4°F), pulse 94/min, respirations 14/min, and oxygen saturation 87% on room air. The patient is given 100% oxygen via nonrebreather mask. Broad-spectrum antibiotics are initiated and bronchoscopic alveolar lavage fluid is sent for culture and sensitivity testing. A diagnosis of hospital-acquired pneumonia is made and the patient is treated with vancomycin for 4 days leading to the resolution of the respiratory symptoms and radiologic resolution of the infiltrate. Subsequently the patient is discharged from the hospital on postoperative day 8 on oral antibiotics and inhaled ipratropium for COPD exacerbations. The surgery resident inputs the patient's hospital course and current medications at the time of transfer in patient's discharge summary and faxes the summary to the patient's PCP. The resident then calls the PCP's office to confirm the receipt of patient's medical record and discharge summary. This hospital's protocol mandates that all discharges be handled in this manner.

Q 13.1: This standardized process of communicating a patient's hospital course with providers in the next setting (e.g., outpatient facilities, PCP) is likely to result in which of the following?

a. Reduction in health care–associated costs
b. Reduction in hospital readmission rates
c. Reduction in hospital-acquired infections
d. Reduction in length of stay times for cholecystectomy

Answers

Case 1 answers

Q 1.1: b. Donabedian model for care quality

This scenario describes a hospital's targeted approach to quality improvement by instituting changes in structures, processes, and outcomes, consistent with the Donabedian model for health care quality. The Donabedian model for care quality utilizes a triad of *structure, process,* and *outcome* as a framework for evaluating the quality of health care.

Structure refers to the setting in which care is delivered, including facilities, equipment, qualifications of providers (e.g., board certification), and administrative systems (e.g., accreditation of hospitals).

Process encompasses the components of care delivery in terms of appropriateness, acceptability, completeness, competence, and coordination.

Outcome refers to the end points of care such as recovery, restoration of function, and survival.

The Donabedian model involves a broader approach to quality measurement (beyond the management of acute illness), incorporating assessments of preventive measures, continuity of care, rehabilitative efforts, the patient–physician relationship, and the economic efficiency of services provided.

The industrial quality management model focuses on the recognition and minimization of variation in the processes of health care delivery. While uniformity helps streamline the delivery of services, it is unable to comprehensively account for factors that impact the overall quality of health care and the determinants of health of the population. Although this question has elements of the industrial quality management (e.g., implementation of the electronic health record system), other changes described are not fully explained by the industrial quality management system.

The quality assurance model focuses on maintaining a high standard of health care services, in accordance with the expectations of the recipients of care. This question elaborates on improvements in all aspects of quality—structures, processes, and outcomes—not just high quality of health care services.

The pay-for-performance (P4P) model incentivizes clinical effectiveness and promotes meeting set minimum requirements for the quality of health care delivery. Although this model focuses on quality improvement and cost effectiveness, minimal emphasis is put on continuum of care, coordination, and structure design, thereby missing important determinants of health.

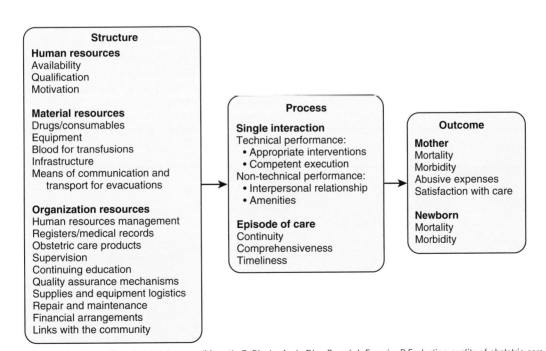

Fig. 1.1 Conceptual framework for the quality of obstetric care. (Morestin F, Bicaba A, de Dieu Sermé J, Fournier P. Evaluating quality of obstetric care in low-resource settings: building on the literature to design tailor-made evaluation instruments—an illustration in Burkina Faso. *BMC Health Serv Res.* 2010;10:20.)

While the P4P model is primarily utilized by payers for determining reimbursement, the Donabedian model still remains the most comprehensive tool for health care quality assessment and improvement.

Suggested further readings

1. Donabedian A. Evaluating the quality of medical care. *Milbank Q.* 2005;83(4):691-729.
2. Laffel G, Blumenthal D. The case for using industrial quality management science in health care organizations. *JAMA.* 1989;262(20):2869-2873.
3. Van Herck P, De Smedt D, Annemans L, Remmen R, Rosenthal MB, Sermeus W. Systematic review: effects, design choices, and context of pay-for-performance in health care. *BMC Health Serv Res.* 2010;10:247.

Case 2 answers

Q 2.1: c. Improvement of the health of the population
In this scenario, the provision of emergent and preventive cardiac services through satellite clinics to a patient population with difficult access to care is expected to improve the overall health of the population.

Q 2.2: a. Improved health of the population, reduced health care costs, enhanced patient experience
The Triple Aim of health care posits that health care delivery should have a primary goal of improving the health of a population and two secondary goals: enhancing the patient experience and reducing the per capita costs of health care.

Q 2.3: c. Risk of health care worker burnout
While the Triple Aim approach aspires to improve the overall health and experience of the patient population, it poses additional workload and expectations on the health care workforce to meet these benchmarks, putting them at an increased risk for burnout and decreased satisfaction with work. Burnout can present as increased cynicism, decreased sense of personal accomplishment, and lack of finding meaning in work. These negative effects on the health care workforce threaten the patient-centered approach outlined in the Triple Aim. Professional burnout among physicians is associated with worse clinical outcomes, increased health care costs, lower patient satisfaction, and lower levels of empathy. Given these detrimental effects of burnout on patient care, it is important to consider measures to improve the work life of those who deliver care. Bodenheimer and Sinsky proposed this as the fourth aim of health care delivery (i.e., the quadruple aim): to improve the work life of health care providers using coordinated team efforts to balance the chasm of expectations with capacity, to provide optimal patient-centered health care.

Suggested further readings

1. Berwick DM, Nolan TW, Whittington J. The Triple Aim: care, health, and cost. *Health Aff (Millwood).* 2008;27(3):759-769.
2. Shanafelt TD, Boone S, Tan L, et al. Burnout and satisfaction with work-life balance among US physicians relative to the general US population. *Arch Intern Med.* 2012;172(18):1377-1385.
3. Bodenheimer T, Sinsky C. From triple to quadruple aim: care of the patient requires care of the provider. *Ann Fam Med.* 2014;12(6):573-576.

Case 3 answers

Q 3.1: b. Computerized prescribing and medication dispensing
This question details one of the most common medical errors—medication dosage errors. A medication error is a failure in the treatment process that leads to, or has the potential to lead to, harm to the patient. The medication error could be an error in choosing the medication, writing the prescription, manufacturing the medication, dispensing the formulation (e.g., wrong drug, wrong dose, wrong label), administering the drug (e.g., wrong route, wrong frequency), and failing to monitor therapy. The use of information technology systems at each of these processes minimizes the likelihood of the occurrence of medication error. An electronic prescription and medication dispensing system is most effective in reducing medication errors.

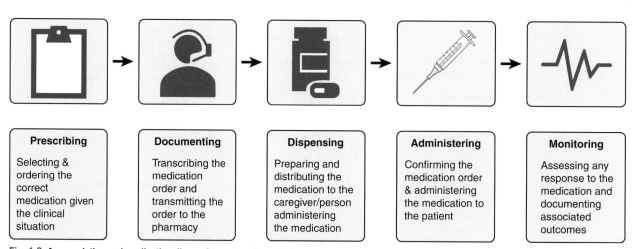

Prescribing	Documenting	Dispensing	Administering	Monitoring
Selecting & ordering the correct medication given the clinical situation	Transcribing the medication order and transmitting the order to the pharmacy	Preparing and distributing the medication to the caregiver/person administering the medication	Confirming the medication order & administering the medication to the patient	Assessing any response to the medication and documenting associated outcomes

Fig. 1.2 A prescription and medication dispensing system for reducing medical errors.

Suggested further readings

1. Agrawal A. Medication errors: prevention using information technology systems. *Br J Clin Pharmacol.* 2009;67(6): 681-686.
2. Aronson JK. Medication errors: what they are, how they happen, and how to avoid them. *QJM.* 2009;102(8): 513-521.
3. *Food and Drug Administration.* Working to reduce medication errors. <https://www.fda.gov/Drugs/ResourcesForYou/Consumers/ucm143553.htm>; 2018 Accessed 01.16.19.

Case 4 answers

Q 4.1: d. All of the above

Workplace design and structure that reflects an alignment of work patterns of employees and the physical settings of the health care facility (e.g., centralized location of supplies, unit layout [radial vs rectangular], decentralized pharmacy systems) have been shown to improve workflow, reduce waiting times, and improve patient satisfaction. The design of a facility can have a significant impact on human performance, patient safety, and experience. Improved facility designs can help reduce staff fatigue and patient and family stress. It can also increase effectiveness in delivering care and subsequently improve outcomes.

Q 4.2: d. Reduction in the noise level

Reduced noise levels in health care settings is associated with positive effects such as reduced perceived work demands, improved quality of care for patients, and better speech intelligibility. Similarly, adequate ventilation and lighting in health care facility design is associated with improved patient and staff safety, including reduced risk for hospital-acquired infections and medication errors. While designing new health care facilities (or renovating old ones) emphasis on the physical structure, environment, and corresponding ergonomic suitability promotes efficient, effective, and safe health care delivery. Awareness of structural factors contributing to patient care and incorporating physicians in the facility design team enables the development of well-designed health care facilities providing highest quality care to patients.

Suggested further readings

1. Blomkvist V. Acoustics and psychosocial environment in intensive coronary care. *Occup Environ Med.* 2005; 62(3):e1.
2. Hendrich AL, Fay J, Sorrells AK. Effects of acuity-adaptable rooms on flow of patients and delivery of care. *Am J Crit Care.* 2004;13(1):35-45.
3. Engbers LH, van Poppel MN, Chin Paw AMJ, van Mechelen W. Worksite health promotion programs with environmental changes: a systematic review. *Am J Prev Med.* 2005;29:61-70.
4. Reiling J. Safe design of healthcare facilities. *Qual Saf Health Care.* 2006;15(suppl 1):i34-i40.
5. Ulrich RS, Zimring C, Zhu X, et al. A review of the research literature on evidence-based healthcare design. *HERD.* 2008;1(3):61-125.

Case 5 answers

Q 5.1: b. Operational capacity of the organization

When there is limited availability of health care providers within an organization, the operational capacity or the total volume of services provided by an organization with the available resources is affected. Responsible resource allocation and workload sharing strives to balance providing excellent patient care with maintaining capacity of the organization. Clinical outcomes and patient satisfaction are the major determinants of *operational effectiveness* of an organization.

Q 5.2: c. Medical errors

Physicians who are overburdened for protracted periods of time are at an increased risk for fatigue and medical errors. While there may be an increase in waiting times for patients and an associated reduced physician–patient interaction time, the risk for medical errors is the most significant negative consequence that may result from excessive physician workload. Increased economic pressure on the health care facilities, inefficient work processes, and physician time constraints can cause physician workload increases beyond safe levels leading to medical errors. The recognition of the effect of excessive workloads on patient safety has led to an increased focus on balancing the operational goals of the health care organization with the availability of health care providers with attempts to increase efficiency via improvements in health care delivery processes such as coordination, automation, and team communication.

Case 6 answers

Q 6.1: c. Physician burnout

Physician burnout is characterized by emotional exhaustion, depersonalization (treating patients as objects), low sense of accomplishment, cynicism, and a lack of a sense of purpose as well as physical exhaustion that does not respond to adequate rest. An alarming number of physicians experience burnout; an estimated 25% to 60% of practicing physicians report symptoms of burnout. The etiology of physician burnout is multifactorial; increased workload, higher stress levels, and decrease in autonomy, combined with a set of unique personality traits (such as compulsiveness, perfectionism, and denial of vulnerability), predispose physicians to burnout. Burnout among physicians is associated with poor quality of care, including decreased patient satisfaction scores and an increased risk for medical errors.

Q 6.2: e. All of the above

To prevent physician burnout, both individual-focused and organization-level interventions are required. The individual-focused interventions that have been shown to reduce the risk of burnout among physicians include mindfulness, stress management training, self-care efforts, exercise training programs, increased social interaction, and engaging in personally fulfilling hobbies and activities. At the organizational level, strategies to reduce the physician workload such as nonphysician staff support, an optimized medical record system, fair productivity targets, and promoting shared decision making help reduce the risk of burnout among physicians.

Q 6.3: c. Better resource allocation

Resource stewardship is a prime concern of health care organizations. Measures directed at assessing time, costs, and rates of services are critical to maintaining the operational efficiency of the organization. When there is a limited pool of physicians, adequate allocation of other health professionals (e.g., physician assistants, nurse practitioners), fair productivity targets, flexible work scheduling, and appropriate distribution of nonclinical roles are useful to prevent overburdening the available physicians. The nature of the relationship between the health care workers and the organization is largely determined by the degree of support and resources provided to the staff by the organization, and its expectations of the staff. While these variables are defined by the organization, they have implications for the culture of the organization, resource/time pressures on the staff, scheduling, and training, which in turn impact health care workers' quality of life and work satisfaction.

Suggested further readings

1. Cowing M, Davino-Ramaya CM, Ramaya K, Szmerekovsky J. Health care delivery performance: service, outcomes, and resource stewardship. *Perm Journal.* 2009;13(4):72-78.
2. Hussey PS, de Vries H, Romley J, et al. A systematic review of health care efficiency measures. *Health Serv Res.* 2009; 44(3):784-805.
3. Shanafelt TD, Sloan JA, Habermann TM. The well-being of physicians. *Am J Med.* 2003;114(6):513-519.
4. Haas JS, Cook EF, Puopolo AL, Burstin HR, Cleary PD, Brennan TA. Is the professional satisfaction of general internists associated with patient satisfaction? *J Gen Intern Med.* 2000;15(2):122-128.
5. Kohn LT, Corrigan JM, Donaldson MS. To Err is Human: Building a Safer Health System: a Report of The Committee on Quality of Health Care in America. *Institute of Medicine.* Washington, DC: National Academies Press; 2000.

Case 7 answers

Q 7.1: a. Never event

This is a classic example of a never event—that is, wrong-site surgery. A never event is a medical error that, with proper safeguards in place, should never occur (e.g., wrong-site surgery, misdiagnosis, wrong procedure). Its definition also includes serious, debilitating adverse events that may have been prevented with adequate care (e.g., pressure ulcers, falls). Health care systems instill processes that facilitate communication between different teams for thorough handoffs and standardize transmission of medical information during points of transition of care to prevent "never events" from occurring.

Q 7.2: f. All of the above

The proper protocol for any surgical procedure includes prior site marking, a time-out before the start of the procedure to confirm site, laterality, and the procedure. Thorough knowledge of the patient's principal medical condition and adequate coordination between teams ensure smooth transition and appropriate communication of clinically relevant facts. All of the options listed are essential for quality health care and to prevent a never event from occurring. These processes are instituted by the hospitals to prevent any medical error and provide the highest quality care to the patient at each level. Furthermore, the hospitals use electronic information systems that record these processes during all aspects of patient interaction with any health care provider, to prevent communication lapses. Additionally, hospitals periodically review all instances of "preventable harm" by evaluating detailed history of the event and identifying opportunities for improvement (e.g., morbidity and mortality conferences).

Q 7.3: d. Hospital

To improve the quality of health care delivered and to strongly deter the occurrence of never events, the Centers for Medicare and Medicaid Services (CMS) has instituted a policy that CMS would not pay any additional costs associated with preventable errors, including never events. Most state and private payers have followed suit and now do not pay for the additional cost associated with a never event. Thus the additional cost is borne by the hospital/health care organization.

Q 7.4: e. All of the above

The National Quality Forum currently lists 29 events as "never events" grouped into seven categories—surgical events, product or device events (e.g., death or serious injury due to contaminated device, air embolism), patient protection events (e.g., patient suicide), care or management events (e.g., serious medication error), environmental events (e.g., electric shock, gas leaks), radiologic events (e.g., introduction of a metallic object into the magnetic resonance imaging [MRI] area), and criminal events (e.g., abduction, battery, sexual assault, or abuse of a patient).

Suggested further readings

1. Michaels RK, Makary MA, Dahab Y, et al. Achieving the National Quality Forum's "never events": prevention of wrong site, wrong procedure, and wrong patient operations. *Ann Surg.* 2007;245(4):526-532.
2. Lembitz A, Clarke TJ. Clarifying "never events and introducing "always events". *Patient Saf Surg.* 2009;3:26.
3. *Agency for Healthcare Research and Quality.* Never events. <https://psnet.ahrq.gov/primers/primer/3/never-events>; 2017 Accessed 05.05.18.

Case 8 answers

Q 8.1: a. Microsystem

A clinical microsystem is defined as a small, functional group of health care professionals who work together on a regular basis to provide care to discrete subpopulations of patients. By optimizing the way small clinical teams or microsystems function, organizations are able to improve transitions of care, coordination, and integration across settings, leading to improved patient safety and care. Each microsystem is a dynamic small-scale clinical enterprise with shared core clinical and business aims, linked processes, and a shared information environment. These microsystems are often embedded into larger systems and organizations referred to as mesosystems and macrosystems. The mesosystems link microsystems together and have them as clinical subunits along the continuum of care, facilitating smooth coordination and transition of care across microsystems. These mesosystems ultimately form the building blocks of the larger health care organization, the macrosystem. For example, an operating room team works together based on shared information (patient's health record), with a common goal to serve the needs of the patient (intraoperative point of care). This team coordinates the patient transition with the postoperative recovery unit team which may be viewed as a separate microsystem for health care services delivery.

Case 9 answers

Q 9.1: d. Skilled nursing facility

This patient with residual deficits is likely going to need long-term care, including nursing, physical therapy, and rehabilitation services, best provided in a long-term care facility such as a skilled nursing facility. Long-term care facilities provide health care, social, and spiritual services to chronically ill patients, typically for 30 days or more. Other facility types include a general hospital, which provides emergency, critical, intensive, and general care to a wide variety of populations, or a specialty hospital, which provides specialized care to specific patient populations such as geriatric patients, cancer patients, patients requiring rehabilitative services, or those requiring specialized psychiatric and psychologic services. Outpatient services refer to health care services provided to those individuals who have not been formally admitted to the facility and usually have a stay of 24 hours or less, including ambulatory care services. The ambulatory care services may be affiliated or connected with a larger hospital (e.g., ambulatory surgery, satellite clinics, observation services) or may be free-standing ambulatory facilities that are not affiliated to a larger hospital or system (e.g., neighborhood health clinics, birthing centers, urgent care centers, industrial health clinics).

Suggested further readings

1. Nelson EC, Batalden PB, Huber TP, et al. Microsystems in health care: part 1. Learning from high-performing frontline clinical units. *Jt Comm J Qual Improv.* 2002;28(9):472-493.
2. Likosky DS. Clinical microsystems: a critical framework for crossing the quality chasm. *J Extra Corpor Technol.* 2014;46(1):33-37.

Case 10 answers

Q 10.1: c. Drug interaction

This patient experienced a significant drop in blood pressure after administration of sublingual nitroglycerin due to a drug interaction with sildenafil—a phosphodiesterase-5 inhibitor—which can cause severe hypotension and death.

During every patient care encounter, it is important to be aware of the patient's current medications to prevent any harmful drug interaction.

Q 10.2: c. Medication reconciliation at admission

Medication reconciliation refers to the formal process of creating a comprehensive, accurate list of a patient's current medications and comparing it to the existing list in the patient record or medication orders. This event could have been prevented by a review of the patient's current medications before administration of the nitroglycerin. To prevent medication errors, most health care facilities include medication reconciliation processes in their systems. Reconciliation is helpful to prevent duplications, omissions, dosing errors, or adverse drug interactions. Recognizing the potential for medication errors, efforts are made to encourage health care providers to perform medication reconciliation at all patient care transitions.

Q 10.3: b. Appropriate documentation of patient's hospital course

Thorough and structured documentation at the time of admission, administration of services, and discharge/transition aids in better communication, coordination, and integration of care across providers. An important component of patient safety is the instillation of practices that promote optimal health care delivery and prevent medical errors. Prior studies report that errors during transitions of care and medication errors are the most common patient safety errors in health care, and on average a hospitalized patient experiences at least one medication error per day. Transitions in care have been recognized as an important area of concern for patient safety, with a potential for medical errors occurring during handoffs. It is important to be aware of pressures that serve as barriers to adequate handoffs.

Suggested further readings

1. Barnsteiner JH. Medication reconciliation. In: Hughes RG, ed. *Patient Safety and Quality: An Evidence-Based Handbook for Nurses.* Rockville, MD: Agency for Healthcare Research and Quality; 2008.
2. Institute of Medicine. *Preventing Medication Errors.* Aspden P, Wolcott J, Bootman JL, Cronenwett LR, eds. Washington, DC: National Academies Press; 2007.
3. Patient Safety Systems Chapter, Sentinel Event Policy and RCA2. *Joint Commission.* <https://www.jointcommission.org/sentinel_event.aspx>; Accessed 11.05.18.
4. Shojania KG, Duncan BW, McDonald KM, Wachter RM, Markowitz AJ. Making health care safer: a critical analysis of patient safety practices. *Evid Rep Technol Assess (Summ).* 2001;(43):i-668.
5. Dvorak SR, McCoy RA, Voss GD. Continuity of care from acute to ambulatory care setting. *Am J Health Syst Pharm.* 1998;55(23):2500-2504.

Case 11 answers

Q 11.1: e. Bundled payment model

The bundled payment/episode of care model provides a single negotiated lump sum amount to be paid for a specified procedure or management of a medical condition (e.g., knee replacement surgery). This model permits reimbursement based on the costs of adhering to clinical standards of care, risk stratification, and allowance for complications. This model benefits from incentivizing efficiency and preventing any unnecessary episodes of care.

Patient-centered medical home (PCMH)

This is a primary care–driven model where a team of health care professionals—the physician, registered nurses (RNs), a case manager, and a medical assistant—coordinate the patient's care across the health care continuum. Under this model, the providers can often negotiate a fee-for-service (FFS) rate increase or a per-member-per-month (PMPM) payment in addition to the standard FFS payments.

Shared savings (One-sided risk)

The shared savings model is similar to the standard FFS structure; however, the shared savings program rewards providers who are able to reduce total health care spending below an expected level set by the payer. It is based on the review of services provided, measured against the estimated medical costs. If there are any savings, the provider is entitled to a share of the savings.

Capitation models

This model is unique in that it sets a payment per patient that a provider receives over a period of time. These are usually in the form of a monthly per-patient fee. These set fees are determined by an actuarial analysis of historic costs of care for the patient population to be covered. Under this model, the provider bears all of the insurance risk for the covered patient and services.

Provider-sponsored health plans (PSHPs)

Under the PSHPs, a provider network—often led by a hospital system—provides health care, and health insurance coverage, thereby assuming the financial risk of insuring that patient population. While the providers are in charge of how care is delivered to patients, or how much is spent on delivering that care in this model, this has been shown to promote higher quality health care at lower costs than the traditional payers plan.

Q 11.2: a. Increase

The traditional fee-for-service model covers the cost of each test, procedure, specialist consultation, and days of hospital stay as utilized, instead of the lump-sum prespecified amount of bundled payments. While the eventual reimbursement may be lower than the amount charged by the hospital, it is usually higher than the reimbursement in a bundled pay model. The reimbursement in the bundled pay incentivizes efficiency over volume, whereas the FFS model prioritizes volume.

Q 11.3: d. Quality of health care

The traditional fee-for-service model in the United States does not incorporate the quality of the services provided and is largely based on the total volume of the services provided. The reimbursement system is in the midst of a major transition—from the traditional volume-based health care models toward value-based health care models, with a goal to better align payment with objective measures of clinical quality. The reimbursements in the value-based health care delivery model are based on patient health outcomes and incentivize provider efforts to help patients improve their health, effectively manage and mitigate harmful effects of chronic diseases, and live healthier lives overall. In addition, these value-based incentives and penalties are dependent upon the quality and performance measures of the health care delivered to the patient population. Health care organizations are transitioning toward a value improvement as a business model by investing in new systems that measure, analyze, and report clinical outcomes as well as costs at the individual patient level. Furthermore, the organizations are investing in creating multidisciplinary teams to integrate and facilitate quality improvement efforts across specialties. These measures are intended to improve the quality of care delivered and subsequently increase reimbursements. While several distinct models for value-based reimbursement currently exist, most fall along a continuum of quality incentive and risk sharing.

Suggested further readings

1. Miller HD. From volume to value: better ways to pay for health care. *Health Aff (Millwood).* 2009;28(5): 1418-1428.
2. Kaplan RS, Witkowski M, Abbott M, et al. Using time-driven activity-based costing to identify value improvement opportunities in healthcare. *J Healthc Manag.* 2014;59(6):399-412.
3. Mayes R. Moving (realistically) from volume-based to value-based health care payment in the USA: starting with Medicare payment policy. *J Health Serv Res Policy.* 2011;16(4):249-251.
4. Porter ME. A strategy for health care reform—toward a value-based system. *N Engl J Med.* 2009;361(2):109-112.

Case 12 answers

Q 12.1: b. Accountable care organization

The provision of care by a group of coordinated health care practitioners, focused on delivering high-quality medical care, along with preventive services while reducing the overall costs at that organization most likely represents the accountable care organization (ACO) model. The development of ACOs is an approach toward better organized care and ensuring accountability among health care providers. ACOs enable the health care administrators, physicians, and other health care professionals to work together effectively to improve cost, while reducing the spending on health care. The ACOs may use a range of reimbursement models, from fee-for-service plans to capitation models. While ACOs currently face challenges due to variation in estimates of average patient costs per annum, this can be minimized by maintaining an adequate target population under their care.

Suggested further readings

1. Fisher ES, Staiger DO, Bynum JPW, Gottlieb DJ. Creating accountable care organizations: the extended hospital medical staff: a new approach to organizing care and

ensuring accountability. *Health Aff (Millwood)*. 2007;26(1):w44-w57.

2. Song Z. Accountable care organizations in the U.S. health care system. *J Clin Outcomes Manag*. 2014;21(8): 364-371.

Case 13 answers

Q 13.1: b. Reduction in hospital readmission rates

Lapses in communication during hospital discharge transitions are associated with increased likelihood of postdischarge complications such as hospital readmissions, medication noncompliance, and injuries. Several federal, state, local, and institutional initiatives emphasize identifying and improving gaps in the transition process. Adequate communication and coordination with the providers in the next setting aids a smooth recovery, prevents hospital readmission, and helps provide adequate follow-up care without a duplication of effort. Health care providers use a combination of methods to communicate important discharge information with the providers in the next setting, including secure emails, faxes, telephone calls, and electronic medical record–based notification applications. Multicomponent care transition provides continuity of care and appropriate follow-up, and prevents postdischarge complications.

Suggested further readings

1. Arora VM, Farnan JM. Care transitions for hospitalized patients. *Med Clin North Am*. 2008;92(2):315-324, viii.
2. Huber TP, Shortell SM, Rodriguez HP. Improving care transitions management: examining the role of accountable care organization participation and expanded electronic health record functionality. *Health Serv Res*. 2017;52(4): 1494-1510.
3. Kripalani S, Jackson AT, Schnipper JL, Coleman EA. Promoting effective transitions of care at hospital discharge: a review of key issues for hospitalists. *J Hosp Med*. 2007;2(5):314-323.

2

Health Care Policy and Economics

Toyin Okanlawon, MD, MPH, Tina R. Shah, MD, MPH

Cases and questions

Q 1.1: Which of the following groups of principal stakeholders is NOT considered one of the classic "four Ps" of health care consumerism?
a. Providers
b. Patients
c. Politicians
d. Public entities
e. Payers

Q 2.1: Political decision making is shaped by the interplay of different actors. The iron triangle describes the independent relationships among which three key actors?
a. Congress, White House, US Department of Health and Human Services
b. Congress, the administration, state governments
c. Congress, the administration, payers
d. Congress, the administration, constituents
e. Congress, the administration, special interest groups

Case 3

Sally Chen is evaluating her health insurance plan options offered by her employer as part of a yearly benefits review. She is 55 years old, has a history of breast cancer, and has no dependents. Last year she was enrolled in Plan A and met her deductible after several hospitalizations and office visits at least once a month with her physicians. She anticipates the same level of health care service utilization in the coming year and is wondering if there is a less expensive plan that will still satisfy her care needs (Table 2.1).

Q 3.1: Premium, deductible, coinsurance, and copay are examples of:
a. Types of health insurance plans
b. Types of health insurance subsidies
c. Cost-sharing mechanisms for the employer
d. Cost-sharing mechanisms for the consumer

Q 3.2: If Sally elects to stay with Plan A, how much money will she have to pay out of pocket for her health care bills before the health insurance plan begins to pay?
a. $35
b. $300
c. $5000
d. None of the above

Q 3.3: Which plan will make it the hardest for Sally to anticipate her out-of-pocket costs for the year?
a. Plan A
b. Plan B
c. Plan C

Table 2.1 Comparison of Health Insurance Plans			
	Plan A (Current)	Plan B	Plan C
Premium	$300/month	$100/month	$500/month
Deductible	$5000	$10,000	$1500
Coinsurance	None	20%/office visit	None
Copay	$35/office visit	None	$20/office visit

Q 3.4: Which plan is the least expensive if no health care is used?
a. Plan A
b. Plan B
c. Plan C

Case 3, continued

Health insurance marketplaces, commonly referred to as health exchanges, are organizations in each state through which individuals, families, and small businesses can purchase medical insurance. Sally also decides to look on her state's health insurance exchange to see how much a plan, comparable to Plan A, would cost if she bought it as an individual rather than through her employer. The premium for an identical plan on the exchange is $700/month.

Q 3.5: Why is the same plan less expensive through her employer?
a. Because employers generally pay a portion of the premium for private health insurance, leaving less for the employee to pay directly
b. Because people who work and are therefore eligible for employer-sponsored health insurance are generally healthier than those who purchase insurance directly on the exchange, so they have lower premiums
c. Because the Affordable Care Act contained a provision to provide tax subsidies to employed consumers to make health insurance more affordable
d. None of the above

Case 4

CareOne, a major insurance provider, is negotiating a contract for reimbursement for services provided by a local primary care practice. For the last ten years, services rendered by the practice resulted in a payment for each service provided. CareOne has just proposed a new payment scheme where the practice is paid a lump sum for each CareOne enrollee seen at the practice to cover all potential services provided over the year. In return for the upfront payment, the practice would agree to care for those particular CareOne enrollees for the year.

Q 4.1: What type of reimbursement arrangement does the practice currently have with CareOne?
a. Pay-for-performance
b. Medicare
c. Accountable care
d. Fee-for-service
e. Capitated

Q 4.2: CareOne contends that the proposed scheme is better than the current one because it promotes the Triple Aim of health reform, defined as:
a. Improving the quality of care, advancing new medical technologies, and reducing the per capita costs of care
b. Improving the quality of care, improving the efficiency of care, and reducing the per capita costs of care
c. Improving the health of populations, improving the experience of care, and reducing the per capita costs of care
d. Improving the health of populations, improving the experience of care, and reducing the amount of public spending on care

Q 4.3: Which of the following statements is true about the new reimbursement scheme?
a. It would increase certainty about how much money CareOne will spend on its enrollees
b. It would increase access to services for CareOne's enrollees
c. It would decrease out-of-pocket costs for enrollees
d. It would improve the experience of care for enrollees

Q 4.4: Which of the following statements is true about the potential impact of the new reimbursement scheme on clinician behavior?
a. It may incentivize delivery of more preventive services such as immunizations and screenings to minimize the need to provide more health care services in the future
b. It may incentivize ordering fewer tests or providing fewer services, even when appropriate, to control costs
c. It would increase clinician autonomy for ordering tests, studies, and medications, which would increase quality of care
d. Both a and b
e. Both a and c

Case 5

For decades, Treble Healthcare, a statewide system comprised of 15 hospitals and 22 community clinics, has relied on fee-for-service reimbursement models. Amy Jacobs, CEO of Treble, has completed her annual performance review with the board of directors. Over the last year, Treble's main competitor, Clef Hospital Corporation, has moved to an entirely value-based model, and now Amy faces pressure from the board to do the same to keep up with the ever-changing marketplace. During next fiscal year, Amy will ask her team to develop bundled payments.

Q 5.1: Which of the following is NOT an objective of value-based health care?
a. Cost containment
b. Generating volume
c. Creating more access
d. Improving patient outcomes

Q 5.2: When designed appropriately, bundled payments should include which of the following component(s):
a. A single payment that covers all the care required to treat a patient's medical condition
b. Being contingent on achieving good, condition-specific outcomes
c. A price that provides a fair margin for delivering effective and efficient care
d. Built-in responsibility for unrelated care
e. All of the above

Case 6

John, an 18-year-old computer science undergraduate student, moved back to his parents' home in Georgia, where he later decided to launch an IT startup. Today, his company has 15 employees and is growing fast. John is relatively healthy and has decided to not obtain his own health insurance. John is ineligible to buy health insurance through his former university but has been able to obtain coverage through his parents' employer.

Q 6.1: Under the Affordable Care Act (ACA), as of 2010, at what age will John no longer be considered a dependent under his parents' insurance plan?

a. 18
b. 21
c. 26
d. 30

Q 6.2: According to the ACA, how many employees must John have on his payroll before he is required to provide his employees with an employer-sponsored health care plan?

a. 20
b. 30
c. 40
d. 50
e. 60

Q 6.3: Recently, both of John's parents retired as elementary school teachers with a full pension plan from the county school system. At age 65, his parents could be eligible for which of the following federally funded programs?

a. AARP (formerly American Association of Retired Persons)
b. Funding for National Institutes of Health Research
c. Medicare
d. Tricare

Q 6.4: An entitlement program guarantees certain benefits to a segment of the population. Common examples of such programs include Social Security, Medicare, and Medicaid. Which of the following is a characteristic of entitlement programs?

a. Mandatory funding that requires annual appropriations
b. Comprises roughly one-third of all federal spending
c. Guarantees funds only for eligible US citizens and permanent residents
d. Funding allocated depends on the number of beneficiaries and the condition of the economy

Case 6, continued

Years later in his late 20s, John can no longer be claimed as a dependent but has remained healthy and maintained a physically active lifestyle. Despite his parents' recommendations, he has decided not to obtain health insurance next year.

Q 6.5: Which of the following is the LEAST accurate statement regarding the individual shared responsibility payment, otherwise known as the individual mandate, which was originally enforced after the Patient Protection and Affordable Care Act was signed into law in 2010?

a. It applies to all individuals who can afford health insurance but choose not to buy
b. It is a key provision of the ACA
c. It requires most individuals to purchase health insurance coverage
d. It requires patients to pay a fee when they file their federal tax return for the year after they don't have coverage

Q 6.6: Which of the following is NOT a requirement for an insurance plan to be certified by the Health Insurance Marketplace?

a. Follow established limits on cost sharing
b. Provide essential health benefits
c. Provide "minimum essential" health coverage
d. Provide (dental/vision control)

Q 6.7: Which of the following types of plans are NOT considered examples of qualifying health coverage?

a. The Children's Health Insurance Program (CHIP)
b. Any health plan purchased through the Health Insurance Marketplace
c. Workers' compensation
d. Medicare Part A or Part C
e. COBRA coverage

Case 7

The creation of Medicaid and Medicare during the Johnson administration (1965) remains one of the most significant legislative achievements in US health reform.

Q 7.1: What characteristic of the Medicaid program served as a lynchpin for the *National Federation of Independent Business v. Sebelius* lawsuit in the post-Affordable Care Act (ACA) era?

a. It was created to provide health coverage for vulnerable populations
b. It was originally funded through federal money with the intent for future private funding through a flat tax on businesses
c. Funding for the program was subject to reappropriation every 10 years
d. Financing for the program was through a combination of federal and state funds

Q 7.2: How did the verdict of *National Federation of Independent Business v. Sebelius* impact the goals of the ACA?

a. It led to an increase in the expected number of newly insured patients, overwhelming hospitals and creating access to care issues
b. It led to a decrease in the expected number of insured patients, increasing financial burden for hospitals that typically provide uncompensated care
c. It increased the amount of federal Medicaid funding to states to support health insurance exchanges
d. It allowed for subsidies for Medicaid to be obtained through state exchanges

Q 7.3: Which state's health care reform law and/or experiment most influenced the approach taken in the ACA?

a. Oregon Health Insurance Experiment
b. Massachusetts Health Connector
c. Vermont's Green Mountain Care
d. Hawaii's Prepaid Health Care Act

Q 7.4: The goals of the Health Insurance Portability and Accountability Act (HIPAA) of 1996 included all the following, EXCEPT:

a. Provision of data privacy and security provisions for safeguarding medical information

b. Protection of health insurance coverage for individuals who lose or change jobs
c. Establishment of national standards for processing electronic health care transactions
d. Increase in bureaucratic burdens on health care providers and institutions

Case 8

Ben, an airplane mechanic for MT Airlines, was injured on the tarmac during a routine engine safety check. He went to the company's health clinic for evaluation. During his intake, he provided important information to the doctor, but it was quickly decided that he had to go to the emergency department for treatment. The clinic does not have an electronic health record and did not bill his employee health plan. Still, Ben remains concerned that his information at the clinic could be shared with his boss.

Q 8.1: In this scenario, which of the following is protected under the HIPAA Privacy Rule?
a. A patient's name, address, birth date, and Social Security number
b. Payment or billing information related to an individual's health
c. A patient's physical or mental health condition
d. All of the above
e. None of the above

Q 8.2: What is the role that congressional authorizing and appropriation committees play in the legislative process?
a. Authorizing committees establish the operational rules for newly passed statutes and modify operational rules for existing statutes, and appropriation committees decide how much federal funding is allocated for discretionary programs in statutes
b. Authorizing committees decide how much federal funding is allocated for discretionary programs in statutes, and appropriation committees establish the operational rules for newly passed statutes and modify operational rules for existing statutes
c. Authorizing committees review and modify bills before they are brought to a vote in the Senate or House of Representatives, and appropriation committees decide how much federal funding is allocated for discretionary programs in statutes
d. Authorizing committees decide how much federal funding is allocated for discretionary programs in statutes, and appropriation committees review and modify bills before they are brought to a vote in the Senate or House of Representatives

Q 8.3: A major component of the Affordable Care Act (ACA) was expanding civil rights protections to consumers. Discrimination in health care based on which of the following was not prohibited prior to the passage of the ACA?
a. Disability
b. Age
c. Gender
d. Race
e. National origin
f. Sexual orientation

Answers

Case 1 answers

Q 1.1: c. Politicians
The US health care ecosystem is extremely complex and is filled with many different stakeholder groups, including payers, providers, patients, regulators, and government agencies. Payers generally refer to entities other than the patient that pay the cost of health services delivered. Although the payer could also be the patient (i.e., beneficiary), it is more common to have third-party payers such as insurance carriers or health plan sponsors (employers, unions, etc.) to be tasked with payments. Providers, including health care professionals and hospitals, have a core mission to deliver health care services to patients, but often differ in their respective bottom line of reimbursement and self-interests. Public entities (e.g., federal government, state public health agencies) regulate and provide health insurance and direct health care services to the population through tax-supported finance programs and venues such as Medicaid/Medicare, public clinics, and hospitals. Choices a, b, d, and e are the four principal stakeholders, or "four Ps," of the health care landscape that can influence political will. Politicians alone, while necessary to create the legislation that regulates the market, are a component of public entities (i.e., not a classic "P").

Case 2 answers

Q 2.1: e. Congress, the administration, special interest groups
The iron triangle is a useful theoretical construct designed to understand the levers of the federal policymaking apparatus. It describes the tightly interdependent relationships among the three major forces that shape decision making: the administration (executive branch), Congress (legislative branch), and interest groups (constituencies). Health care providers are impacted directly by the policymaking process or lack thereof. The iron triangle describes how regulations imparted through funding mechanisms can impact care on the front lines. For example, over the last decade, health care providers have sometimes had to explain to patients that they are unable to receive recommended or needed treatment because of drug shortages. The Food and Drug Administration and other regulatory agencies have collaborated with pharmaceutical companies to address these shortages. A more general example is the federal self-referral statue called the Stark law, which prohibits a provider from referring Medicare and Medicaid patients for designated health services if the provider (or an immediate family member) has a financial relationship with the entity to which the patient is referred. For example, a provider cannot send a patient who sustained a head injury after a fall for an image (i.e., magnetic resonance image [MRI], computed tomography [CT]) at a facility that he or she owns.

Case 3 answers

Q 3.1: d. Cost-sharing mechanisms for the consumer

Cost sharing occurs when the patient pays a portion of health care costs not covered by health insurance. These out-of-pocket payments include deductibles, coinsurance, copayments, and similar charges, but not premiums, balance billing amounts for nonnetwork providers, or the cost of noncovered services. In the United States, rising costs have led employers to increase the cost-sharing provisions of their health plans. Consumer-driven health plans, although a small share of the health insurance market, include greater consumer cost sharing and have become more prevalent. Although cost sharing is designed to reduce the utilization of unnecessary health care services and increase the cost consciousness of consumers, it may discourage people from using necessary health care and can be inequitable for the very sick and those with low incomes. A premium is the price paid by the consumer to have the insurance plan, regardless of whether health care is utilized. It is generally paid in monthly installments using pretax dollars. A deductible is the amount of a health care bill that the enrollee must pay before the insurance plan begins to pay. In addition to the premium and deductible, insurance plans generally use coinsurance and copays as cost-sharing mechanisms. Coinsurance is the percentage of a health care bill the enrollee must pay after the deductible amount has been met, and a copay is a flat fee that the enrollee must pay based on location of care (e.g., office visit or emergency department visit) for each instance of care received. A copayment may also be necessary when patients visit their primary care physician, even if the deductible has been met.

Q 3.2: c. $5000

This question is asking about the plan's deductible or out-of-pocket expense. For Plan A, the deductible is $5000. Once Sally pays for health care bills up to the deductible amount, her insurance will start to pay for part of the bills. Note that the deductible is not the total out-of-pocket maximum that an enrollee will have. For example, after Sally has met her deductible of $5000, any subsequent office visits will still require her to pay $35 a visit. Insurance plans also have a defined maximum out-of-pocket allowance per benefit year. This maximum allowance is important to consider when choosing a specific health plan. For example, an insurance company may have a maximum out-of-pocket allowance of $50,000, thereby limiting the patient from paying beyond this cap in a given year.

Q 3.3: b. Plan B

Out of the listed cost-sharing mechanisms for the insurance plans, coinsurance is the only mechanism that utilizes a percentage rather than a flat fee. Because patients have little control over the charges in their health care bills, Plan B, which contains coinsurance, would make estimating out-of-pocket yearly costs the most challenging.

Q 3.4: b. Plan B

This question is asking what a premium is, which is the only cost an enrollee has regardless of whether health care is utilized. The plan with the lowest premium is Plan B.

Q 3.5: a. Because employers generally pay a portion of the premium for private health insurance, leaving less for the employee to pay directly

Private health insurance that is sponsored by employers is the most common form of health insurance. In 2016, private health insurance coverage continued to be more prevalent than government coverage, at 67.5% and 37.3%, respectively. Of the subtypes of health insurance coverage, employer-based insurance covered 55.7% of the population for some or all of the calendar year, followed by Medicaid (19.4%), Medicare (16.7%), direct purchase (16.2%), and military coverage (4.6%). In employer-based plans, the premium is partially paid by employers as part of employee benefits, leaving a lesser amount to be paid by the enrollee directly. For example, the full insurance premium for Sally in her current situation may be $450. She pays $300 while her employer pays $150. While the premium amount that Sally is responsible for from the employer-sponsored plan was lower than the premium of the plan on the exchange, sometimes that is not the case. The pool of employees in a company may have a wider set of health care needs. Health care complexity is often more heterogeneous than for those who purchase insurance on the exchanges, thus increasing the difficulty for insurers to estimate costs. As a result, insurers may set higher premiums and utilize other methods of cost sharing, which increase costs to the employee (policyholder) and their employers.

Suggested further readings

1. United States Census Bureau. Health insurance coverage in the United States: 2016. <https://www.census.gov/library/publications/2017/demo/p60-260.html>; 2017 Accessed 21.08.18.
2. Askin E, Moore N, Shankar V, Peck W. *The Health Care Handbook: A Clear and Concise Guide to the United States Health Care System*. 2nd ed. St. Louis: Academic Publishing Services, Washington University School of Medicine; 2014.
3. Blumenthal D, Morone J. *The Heart of Power: Health and Politics in the Oval Office*. Los Angeles: University of California Press; 2010.

Case 4 answers

Q 4.1: d. Fee-for-service

The current reimbursement model is fee-for-service. The practice receives payment from CareOne each time a service (e.g., procedure or visit) is provided. This model is desirable in that the financial arrangement is simple yet may have the unintended consequence of incentivizing clinicians to provide unnecessary care because they will receive more pay from "doing more."

Q 4.2: c. Improving the health of populations, improving the experience of care, and reducing the per capita costs of care

The Triple Aim is a term described by the Institute for Healthcare Improvement containing the three core aims of health reform: improving the health of populations, improving the experience of care, and reducing per capita costs of care. While the model serves as a guiding light for policymakers, in practice the complexity of our health care system makes it challenging to achieve all three aims in a given policy.

Q 4.3: a. It would increase certainty about how much money CareOne will spend on its enrollees

The newly proposed reimbursement scheme is an example of a capitated model, where the fee for services provided is based on a flat fee per patient. It was developed by insurers as a response to control rising costs of health care. From the patient perspective, capitation is advantageous because it incentivizes clinicians to prioritize preventive care to minimize the need for costly care in the future, such as hospitalizations. Research on the impact of capitation on patient experience, out-of-pocket costs, and access to care has been mixed. Therefore, while choices b, c, and d are plausible, they are not fully substantiated.

Q 4.4: d. Both a and b

a. It may incentivize delivery of more preventive services such as immunizations and screenings to minimize the need to provide more health care services in the future.

b. It may incentivize ordering fewer tests or providing fewer services even when appropriate to control costs.

This question highlights the complexity of assessing the impact of various reimbursement models and the complexity of relationships between providers, patients, and insurers. While the original intent of the capitated model is to help insurers manage the increasing costs of labor and goods in health care, it was also theorized to have positive impact on patient care by incentivizing clinicians to deliver more preventive care (choice a). However, given that physicians and other health care professionals face greater financial risk because they may be providing more care than covered by the capitated payment received, this model could conceivably influence clinicians to provide less care or withhold necessary care to patients to control costs (choice b). Choice c is incorrect because value-based care is designed to encourage coordination among providers to follow evidence-based guidelines to achieve better health outcomes.

Case 5 answers

Q 5.1: b. Generating volume

Under the fee-for-service model, providers are paid for services performed. This has led to some providers ordering more tests, performing more procedures, and managing more patients in order to get paid more. Costs are determined by what commercial payers will pay in the private market and a percentage of what Medicare would have paid for similar services. Rates for services are also unbundled, meaning each service is paid for separately and providers are paid retrospectively for services delivered based on bill charges or annual fee schedules. Health care policy experts believe the US reliance on this fragmented payment scheme and its incentives to do more, despite suboptimal outcomes, has been the main culprit driving rising health care costs. To drive down health care costs and improve outcomes, the Centers for Medicare and Medicaid Services (CMS) has introduced value-based care models. Value-based health care ties payments for care delivery to the quality of care provided and rewards providers for both efficiency and effectiveness. Of the options listed, value-based health care has been shown to achieve cost containment, more access, greater patient engagement, and improved outcomes.

Q 5.2: e. All of the above

Value-based health care reimbursement models include accountable care organizations (ACOs), bundled payments, and patient-centered medical homes. Bundled payments share the following five main characteristics:

  i. A single payment that covers all the care required to treat a patient's medical condition
  ii. Contingent on achieving good, condition-specific outcomes, including care guarantees
  iii. Risk adjusted or covering a defined patient group in terms of complexity
  iv. Specified limits of responsibility for unrelated care and stop loss provisions to mitigate against outliers and catastrophic events
  v. A price that provides a fair margin for delivering effective and efficient care

Bundled payment, or episode-based payment, is a single payment for services provided for an entire episode of care (choice a). Providers are collectively reimbursed for the expected costs to treat a specific condition that may include several physicians, settings of care, and procedures (choice b). If a patient undergoes surgery, CMS would combine the set payment to the hospital, surgeon, and anesthesiologist, rather than paying each one separately. The bundled payment is determined on historical prices for delivering effective and efficient care (choice c). The onus is on each member to coordinate and deliver outcomes for the condition; for purposes of the bundled payment itself, providers are not responsible for any unrelated care that may occur or catastrophic events. For example, if a patient who undergoes a total knee replacement is discharged home and the next day gets hits by a car and needs another knee surgery, his total knee replacement bundle would not be expected to pay for the treatment of the injury from this accident.

Suggested further readings

1. Porter ME, Teisberg EO. *Redefining Health Care: Creating Value-Based Competition on Results*. Brighton, MA: Harvard Business Review Press; 2006.
2. Porter ME, Kaplan RS. How to pay for health care. *Harv Bus Rev.* 2016;94(7-8):88-100.

Case 6 answers

Q 6.1: c. 26

Prior to the Affordable Care Act (ACA), many health plans and insurers could remove children from their parents' coverage because of their age, whether or not they were a student and regardless of where they lived. The ACA requires plans and issuers that offer dependent child coverage to make the coverage available until the adult child reaches the age of 26. Many parents and their children who worried about losing health coverage after graduating from college now have extended coverage, which applies regardless of the child's marital status. This rule applies to all plans in the individual market and employer-sponsored plans.

Q 6.2: d. 50

The employer mandate requires employers with 50 or more employees to offer affordable health insurance or pay a penalty. Employers with fewer than 50 full-time employees are not subject to tax penalties for not offering health insurance coverage. Although if an employer of this size does provide health insurance, it may be eligible for tax credits.

Q 6.3: c. Medicare

Medicare is available for people age 65 or older. It also provides health insurance to younger people with some disability statuses, as determined by the Social Security Administration (SSA), and to people with end-stage renal disease and amyotrophic lateral sclerosis (Lou Gehrig disease).

You may qualify for Medicare before age 65 if any of the following occur:

- You are disabled and have received disability benefits from the SSA or certain Railroad Retirement Board disability benefits for at least 2 years
- You have Lou Gehrig disease
- You have end-stage renal disease

Medicare is funded by a payroll tax, premiums, surtaxes from beneficiaries, and general revenue. AARP, Inc. (choice a) is a US-based interest group that focuses on the elderly, especially on how they can continue to live well after retirement. In 2016, it had a membership of over 37 million people. Tricare provides civilian health benefits for US Armed Forces military personnel, military retirees, and their dependents, including some members of the Reserve Component (choice d). Medicare coverage is the same for people who qualify based on disability as for those who qualify based on age. For those who are eligible, the full range of Medicare benefits is available. Coverage includes certain hospitals, nursing homes, and home health, physician, and community-based services. The health care services do not have to be related to the individual's disability to be covered.

Q 6.4: d. Funding allocated depends on the number of beneficiaries and the condition of the economy

There are three different types of federal funding mechanisms to implement programs and enact legislation: discretionary funding, mandatory funding, and tax spending. Entitlement programs (e.g., Medicare, Social Security) are services granted to eligible Americans that are guaranteed through direct or mandatory federal spending. Mandatory funding does not require annual appropriations (choice a) and can only be changed by modifying the underlying authorizing statute—an unprecedented action given the longstanding benefits to constituents. In contrast to discretionary funding, about two-thirds of all federal spending funds these

"entitlement" services (choice b). Since the mid-1980s, such programs have accounted for more than half of all federal spending. While most programs such as Social Security were designed for individual citizens or residents, beneficiaries could also be businesses or local governments. The importance of entitlement programs cannot be overstated despite certain challenges.

Q 6.5: a. It applies to all individuals who can afford health insurance but choose not to buy

The individual mandate is a core component of the ACA (choice b). If individuals who can afford health insurance choose not to buy it, they may be required to pay a fee called the individual shared responsibility payment. The fee is owed for any month an individual, his or her spouse, or tax dependents do not have qualifying health coverage. In some cases individuals qualify for an exemption from the requirement to have insurance and thus do not have to pay the fee. It is important to note that exemptions exist, despite the financially punitive nature of the mandate itself. Such exemptions may include but are not limited to the following: coverage that is considered unaffordable, short coverage gap for less than 3 consecutive months during the year, citizens living abroad, and incarcerated individuals. If someone is unemployed and between jobs, the penalty is prorated to cover only the uninsured months. An individual is not assessed a penalty for a gap in coverage less than 3 months. This is called a "short gap." However, you are only allowed one short gap per year. Herein lies an important point. Laws often have caveats or exceptions that provide a bit of leeway.

Q 6.6: d. Provide (dental/vision control)

A health plan that is certified by the Health Insurance Marketplace provides essential health benefits (i.e., meets minimum essential coverage) and follows established limits on cost sharing (including deductibles, copayments, and out-of-pocket maximum amounts). Cited examples include individual plans such as those listed on the exchange, employer-sponsored plans, and government-sponsored coverage plans (Medicare, Medicaid, and CHIP).

Q 6.7: c. Workers' compensation

"Qualifying" affordable coverage meets the minimum essential coverage, thereby avoiding the penalty. Essential health benefits fall into 10 categories:

1. Ambulatory patient services (outpatient services)
2. Emergency services
3. Hospitalization
4. Maternity and newborn care
5. Mental health and substance use disorder services, including behavioral health treatment
6. Prescription drugs
7. Rehabilitative services (those that help patients acquire, maintain, or improve skills necessary for daily functioning) and devices
8. Laboratory services
9. Preventive and wellness services and chronic disease management
10. Pediatric services, including oral and vision care

The Consolidated Omnibus Budget Reconciliation Act (COBRA) gives workers and their families who lose their health benefits the right to choose to continue group health benefits provided by their group health plan for limited periods of time under certain circumstances such as voluntary or involuntary job loss, reduction in the hours worked, transition between jobs, death, divorce, and other life events. Qualified individuals may be required to pay the entire premium for coverage up to 102% of the cost to the plan (choice e). There are some health plans that may pay for specific medical services but do not qualify as coverage. Examples may include coverage only for vision care or dental care, workers' compensation (choice c), coverage only for a specific disease or condition, and plans that offer only discounts on medical services.

Suggested further reading

1. McDonough JE. The United States health system in transition. *Health Syst Reform*. 2015;1(1):39-51.

Case 7 answers

Q 7.1: d. Financing for the program was through a combination of federal and state funds

The financing structure for Medicaid created a point of contention leading to the 2012 lawsuit *National Federation of Independent Business v. Sebelius*. Medicaid is jointly financed by federal funding that is matched to state funds for providing health coverage to vulnerable populations. This structure was modeled after the 1960 Kerr-Mills legislation for Medical Assistance to the Aged. A major provision of the Affordable Care Act (ACA) was to decrease the number of uninsured by expanding Medicaid. The federal government incentivized states to spend more on Medicaid by promising a large share of funding to match state dollars for year 1, with a plan for a gradual decrease in federal support to states over several years. Twenty-six states in this lawsuit challenged this part of the ACA, claiming that federal government was overly coercive of the states and was threatening to cut all federal funds for Medicaid (including existing) if they did not comply with expansion of the program. While choice A is correct, it was not the point of contention which led to the lawsuit. Choices b and c are incorrect.

Q 7.2: b. It led to a decrease in the expected number of insured patients, increasing financial burden for hospitals that typically provide uncompensated care

This Supreme Court case questioned the legality of the federal government to mandate state expansion of Medicaid. The court ultimately decided that mandating Medicaid expansion was unconstitutional, allowing states to choose whether they wanted to expand and ensuring that the current federal funding received for Medicaid would not be revoked. As of April 2018, 18 states had not expanded Medicaid. Compared to estimates by policymakers when the ACA was devised, this significantly reduced the actual number of newly insured patients. To offset increased funding for Medicaid expansion, the

ACA removed Disproportionate Share Hospital payments, which are federal funds to support hospitals that provide higher proportions of uncompensated care. Because there was a smaller reduction in the number of uninsured patients than predicted, hospitals now face an increased financial burden of having to care for these uninsured patients without getting their previous federal compensation.

Q 7.3: b. Massachusetts Health Connector

Hawaii's Prepaid Health Care Act of 1974 (choice d) expanded health insurance coverage by mandating that employers provide health insurance to employees working at least 20 hours per week. Although the ACA has a different threshold for the employer mandate, Hawaii's template was an early precursor to one of the major components of today's law. In 2011 Vermont created the now abandoned state-funded and -managed insurance pool that would provide near universal coverage to residents with the expectation that it would reduce health care spending. However, within 3 short years, the Green Mountain Care plan (choice c) proved too costly to sustain without a significant tax increase. The experience illustrated the difficulty of achieving major health care system transformation in an affordable, budget-sensitive way. The Oregon Health Insurance Experiment (choice a) is a landmark study of the effect of expanding public health insurance on health care use, health outcomes, financial strain, and well-being of low-income adults. It uses an innovative randomized controlled design to evaluate the impact of Medicaid in the United States. The ACA was most influenced by the Massachusetts 2006 health care law, an act providing access to affordable, quality, accountable health care. Among the law's provisions were a mandate that nearly all state residents obtain a minimum level of insurance coverage; sliding-scale subsidized health coverage for individuals with incomes below 300% of the federal poverty level (FPL), with fully subsidized coverage for those below 150% of the FPL; establishment of the Massachusetts Health Connector, an insurance exchange where consumers can select from private, subsidized, and free health insurance plans depending on their income and eligibility; and a requirement that employers with more than 10 full-time employees provide health insurance. The Massachusetts Health Connector (choice b) became the template for the health insurance exchanges. Other components of Massachusetts state law were also adopted in the federal plan. Some of the architects behind this landmark state legislation were also authors of the ACA.

Q 7.4: d. Increase in bureaucratic burdens on health care providers and institutions

The Health Insurance Portability and Accountability Act of 1996—perhaps most well known for its privacy rule that regulated the restricted use and disclosure of protected health information (PHI) (choice a)—had two main goals: to provide continuous health insurance coverage for workers who lose or change their job (choice b) and to reduce (not increase) the administrative burdens and cost of health care by standardizing the electronic transmission of administrative and financial transactions (choice d). Other goals included combating abuse, fraud, and waste in health insurance and health care delivery and improving access to long-term care services and health insurance. One important result of HIPAA is the rapid expansion of health information technologies and creating national standards for processing data (choice c).

Case 8 answers

Q 8.1: c. A patient's physical or mental health condition

Protected health information (PHI) under US law is any information about health status, provision of health care, or payment for health care that is created or collected by a covered entity (or a business associate of a covered entity) and can be linked to a specific individual. Covered entities are defined by the regulation as a health plan or health care providers. Of note, there are a variety of methods to de-identify such information but the discussion would be outside the scope of this question. An onsite health clinic at your place of employment may be another example of what the HIPAA Privacy Rule calls a "hybrid" entity. This depends on whether the health clinic transmits information electronically and engages in standard transactions under HIPAA's electronic data interchange rule (e.g., if the clinic bills an employee's health plan). If so, the records maintained by the health clinic are subject to the same protections that apply to other covered entities. However, if the clinic does not transmit information electronically or bill your employer, it would be specifically excluded from HIPAA's protections.

Q 8.2: a. Authorizing committees establish the operational rules for newly passed statutes and modify operational rules for existing statutes, and appropriation committees decide how much federal funding is allocated for discretionary programs in statutes

Legislation in the United States is a complicated process. After a bill is passed by both the House of Representatives and Senate and signed by the president, it formally becomes known as a statute. Statutes are legislative law and are written in a legal language much like the code that underlies a computer program. To fully implement a law, operational rules or an administrative law must be written and funding allocated. Both chambers of Congress have parallel authorizing and appropriation committees, which work together. The authorizing committees (e.g., the Senate Health, Education, Labor, and Pensions Committee in the case of health-related statutes) review the legislative law and craft the administrative law to operationalize the statute. Appropriation committees in contrast are responsible for deciding the amount of funding to be allocated for any discretionary programs outlined in the statute. The appropriations work is especially important, because if a committee chooses not to complete the process of allocating funds then the law is not put into effect. This is a method used to delay or prevent implementation of part of a statute. In the Affordable Care Act, lack of appropriations prevented creation of a National Healthcare Workforce Commission, even though it is part of the passed legislation.

Q 8.3: c. Gender

Prior to the passage of the ACA, gender discrimination was not prohibited in health care and health services and was typically targeted toward women. Before ACA regulations went into effect, a study conducted by the National Women's Law Center showed that women were paying $1 billion more in premiums than men each year for the same health plan purchased on the individual insurance market. Gender rating also occurred in insurance plans offered through employers. For example, small businesses that primarily employed women, such as hair salons or nonprofits, were charged higher rates by insurers than those in male or mixed sex businesses. In addition to higher costs for insurance coverage, the ACA prohibits denying women health insurance coverage for preexisting conditions that either can only affect women or disproportionately affect women, such as pregnancy and sexual assault. Further, the ACA also mandates insurers cover medications and services that particularly apply to women, including contraceptives, breastfeeding counseling, and cervical cancer screening. Sexual minorities are still not protected from discrimination under any federal health statute.

3

Clinical Informatics and Technology

Claude J. Pirtle, MD

Cases and questions

Case 1

Mr. Jason Sanders is a 75-year-old Caucasian male who presents to a clinic one afternoon. He is a new patient who recently moved to this town from a city on the west side of the state. He states that his past medical issues include high cholesterol, hypertension, anxiety, and dementia. The patient brings a list of five medications—lisinopril, simvastatin, alprazolam, hydrocodone-acetaminophen, and donepezil hydrochloride. The patient states he received a few immunizations at his prior primary care physician's clinic, but he does not remember the names of the injections. The patient states he feels well today, but sometimes he feels as if he has forgotten what he has done earlier in the day.

Q 1.1: Which of the following technologies would be most appropriate to use in this context to receive a list of his prior immunizations?
a. Health information exchange
b. Computerized physician order entry
c. Telemedicine
d. Clinical decision support
e. All of the above

Q 1.2: Clinical decision support (CDS) offers a multitude of opportunities to improve the quality of data collected, including data review and assessment. Which of the following is not one of the "five rights" of CDS that could be used to guide the creation of a CDS intervention?
a. The information should be presented through the correct channel
b. The information should be recently edited by a peer
c. The information should appear at the right time in the workflow

d. The information should be presented to the right person
e. The information should be in the correct format

Q 1.3: What is the name of the federal program created by the Health Information Technology for Economic and Clinical Health Act of 2009 (HITECH) that established objectives for providers to meet, to demonstrate appropriate use of their electronic health records (EHRs) and receive an incentive payment?
a. Certified Electronic Health Record Systems
b. Meaningful Use
c. Health Insurance Portability and Accountability Act
d. Fast Health Care Interoperability Resources
e. Medicare Access and CHIP Reauthorization Act

Q 1.4: Which of the following would be an advantage to using an electronic health record (EHR) system?
a. Enabling safer and more reliable prescribing
b. Promoting more legible, accurate, and complete documentation
c. Enabling quick access to records for improved, coordinated care
d. Providing up-to-date and complete information about patients at the point of care
e. All of the above

Q 1.5: When an EHR system queries a state immunization database exchange or other central repository, which of the following data standards are most likely to be used in the exchange of data?
a. Health Level 7
b. Digital Imaging and Communications in Medicine
c. Hypertext Markup Language
d. Current Procedural Terminology
e. Cascading Style Sheets

Q 1.6: The physician notices that Mr. Sanders's medication list contains an opioid medication named hydrocodone-acetaminophen. What is the name of the database Mr. Sanders's physician would access to find out more information about this drug's prescription, such as the amount of medication dispensed and the prescriber of the medication?

a. Opioid Abuse Monitoring Directory
b. Pharmacist Real-Time Monitoring Program
c. Substance Abuse Collection Index
d. Prescription Drug Monitoring Program
e. Federal Drug Database Program

Case 2

Mr. Sanders's spouse arrives and states that he was recently admitted to a local hospital for pneumonia. The patient's spouse states he was in the hospital for about 3 days. She doesn't remember what antibiotics he was on at that time but states he did have a lot of blood drawn and a few chest X-rays.

Q 2.1: Health care information—including notes, immunizations, diagnosis codes, and a myriad of other variables—add up to an enormous amount of data. A data warehouse is a database allowing data to be extracted from a larger dataset or multiple datasets. Which of the following is a benefit of extracting the data of interest into a smaller dataset?

a. Allows for data analysis to process faster than if the analytics were done on the full set of data
b. Data warehouses are only made up of financial data
c. Frequent queries can be done on the database for near real-time data
d. Both a and c
e. All of the above

Q 2.2: When entering Mr. Sanders's diagnosis into the chart, which of the following coding standards would the physician use in her EHR to report the appropriate diagnosis?

a. Fast Health Interoperability Resources (FHIR)
b. Logical Observation Identifiers Names and Codes (LOINC)
c. RxNorm
d. International Classification of Diseases (ICD)
e. Gold Standard Disease Databank

Q 2.3: The physician has access to Mr. Sanders's chart at his hospital through a health information exchange (HIE). The physician is able to view all of Mr. Sanders's laboratory and radiology results as well as his past discharge summary and other notes. Which of the following is an example of an unstructured data element that can be found in Mr. Sanders's chart?

a. Discharge summary
b. Laboratory result
c. Vital sign
d. Patient demographics
e. All of the above

Q 2.4: Mr. Sanders's chest X-ray is stored on a hospital's Picture Archival and Communication System (PACS) in a format called Digital Imaging and Communication in Medicine (DICOM). Which of the following is the benefit to storing all radiology images in this standard format?

a. The DICOM standard dictates a consistent set of rules for the communication of digital images

b. The DICOM standard is only used in the United States
c. DICOM is an extremely adaptable standard
d. Both a and c
e. All of the above

Q 2.5: Although EHRs provide a number of benefits to a patient's overall care, disadvantages also exist. Which of the following is an advantage to the current use of an EHR?

a. Increased physician burnout
b. Improved coordinated care
c. Reduction in productivity
d. Less time for face-to-face patient care
e. All of the above

Case 3

During the interview, the physician asks Mr. Sanders about his family history. Mr. Sanders's spouse states that his younger brother was recently diagnosed with amyotrophic lateral sclerosis (ALS). Mr. Sanders's spouse states he was entered into a clinical registry that should have all of his information.

Q 3.1: Which of the following is true of a clinical data registry?

a. A clinical data registry is required to be implemented at each center that treats a specific disease (e.g., ALS)
b. Clinical data registries do not provide helpful information to improve a patient's care
c. A clinical data registry structures data in a suboptimal way, which does not allow research to be performed very easily
d. A clinical data registry is a record of the health status of a patient and the health care he or she has received over a period of time
e. Both a and c

Q 3.2: Over the past few years, health care technology has continued to improve, offering a more robust experience for each patient in many aspects, including quality of life. Which of the following is a technology that has helped improve health care?

a. Telehealth services
b. Electronic health records (EHRs)
c. Mobile technologies
d. Improved connectivity of physicians and patients
e. All of the above

Q 3.3: Which of the following fields of informatics could be best described as "informatics applied in health care or individual health setting"?

a. Public health informatics
b. Clinical informatics
c. Imaging informatics
d. Translational bioinformatics
e. None of the above

Case 4

After completing Mr. Sanders's office visit, the physician writes a prescription for a blood pressure cuff and refills two of his medications using electronic prescribing. The physician asks Mr. Sanders to follow up via telemedicine in 2 weeks.

Q 4.1: Which of the following is considered a "medical device" according to the US Food and Drug Administration (FDA)?
a. A tongue depressor
b. Programmable pacemaker
c. X-ray machine
d. Surgical laser device
e. All of the above

Q 4.2: When classifying a "medical device" with the FDA, the classification depends on the intended use of the device and on the indications for use. In addition, the classification is based on the risk the device poses to the patient and/or user. Which of the following classes would include the devices with the most significant risk?
a. Class I
b. Class II
c. Class III
d. Class IV
e. None of the above

Q 4.3: The physician's office schedules a follow-up visit with Mr. Sanders using a new telehealth system. Which of the following is true of telemedicine use?
a. Improves patient access to care
b. All private and public insurers will reimburse telemedicine visits
c. Improves cost efficiency and patient satisfaction
d. Both a and c
e. None of the above

Q 4.4: Which of the following acts required the Department of Health and Human Services to develop privacy and security regulations to protect certain health information?
a. Employee Retirement Income Security Act (ERISA)
b. Medicare Drug, Improvement, and Modernization Act
c. Consolidated Omnibus Budget Reconciliation Act
d. Health Information Technology for Economic and Clinical Health Act (HITECH)
e. Health Insurance Portability and Accountability Act (HIPAA)

Q 4.5: Which of the following techniques could be used to help forecast the potential of Mr. Sanders being readmitted to the hospital within 30 days?
a. Machine learning
b. Data mining
c. Predictive modeling
d. Both a and c
e. All of the above

Case 5

Mr. Sanders's wife is interested in a new technology called "mobile health." Mr. Sanders's wife asks his physician if he would be a good candidate to use some of the mobile health devices.

Q 5.1: Which of the following is true regarding the use of mobile health technology?
a. Increased ability to reach underserved populations
b. All mobile health applications are regulated by the FDA
c. Decreased medication compliance
d. Both a and c
e. All of the above

Q 5.2: The physician is able to access some of Mr. Sanders's data via a health information exchange (HIE). Which of the following is not an example of an HIE architecture?
a. Direct HIE model
b. Decentralized HIE model
c. Centralized HIE model
d. Indexed HIE model
e. All of the above are examples of an HIE architecture

Q 5.3: When accessing Mr. Sanders's data via an office-based desktop computer, which of the following is a data protection method used to help keep the data confidential and preserve the data's integrity whenever transferring data from one location to another?
a. Structured query
b. Distributed migration
c. Authentication
d. Encryption
e. Both c and d

Q 5.4: When accessing Mr. Sanders's chart, the physician realizes that the chart was recently accessed by another clinician in the office. Which of the following terms best describes the "extra" data, such as the time this physician accessed the record?
a. Metadata
b. Administrative data
c. Enterprise data
d. Adaptive data
e. Both a and c

Q 5.5: When entering prescriptions for two medications, the physician takes advantage of computerized provider order entry (CPOE). Which of the following is a benefit that CPOE offers?
a. CPOE allows quicker transmission of orders to the radiology department and pharmacy
b. CPOE allows the ability to recommend alternative tests, treatments, or medications in the workflow of ordering
c. It reduces errors in medication prescriptions
d. Both a and c
e. All of the above

Q 5.6: One Meaningful Use Stage 2 core objective required that patients have electronic access to their health information. Which of the following could Mr. Sanders use to access and view his health information from home?
a. Patient portal
b. Patient exchange
c. Designated patient gateway
d. Both a and c
e. All of the above

Answers

Case 1 answers

Q 1.1: a. Health information exchange
A health information exchange (HIE) can be described in two separate ways. According to the Office of the

National Coordinator for Health Information Technology, an HIE, when used as a verb, is the appropriate and confidential electronic exchange of clinical information among authorized organizations such as physician offices and hospital systems. An HIE, when used as a noun, is an organization with agreed-upon operational and business rules that provides services to enable the electronic and secure sharing of health-related information. An example of an HIE used as a noun would be a state-based health information exchange that allows the transfer of documents such as health summaries or continuity of care documents.

Suggested further readings

1. What is health information exchange? <https://www.healthit.gov/faq/what-health-information-exchange>; 2017 Accessed 25.04.18.
2. American Medical Association. Health information exchange interoperability. <https://www.ama-assn.org/practice-management/digital/health-information-exchange-interoperability>; 2018 Accessed 30.04.18.

Q 1.2: b. The information should be recently edited by a peer

The Office of the National Coordinator for Health Information Technology defines clinical decision support (CDS) as "providing clinicians, staff, patients, or other individuals with knowledge and person-specific information, intelligently filtered or presented at appropriate times, to enhance health and health care." The "five rights" of CDS can be used whenever planning to implement a CDS intervention at an institution. They serve as a scheme to achieve CDS-supported improvements in a desired health care arena. The "five rights" can be communicated as giving the right information to the right person in the right CDS intervention format, through the right channel, and in the right workflow.

Suggested further readings

1. Campbell R. The five rights of clinical decision support: CDS tools helpful for meeting meaningful use. *J AHIMA*. 2013;84(10):42-47.
2. Office of the National Coordinator for Health Information Technology. Clinical decision support. <https://www.healthit.gov/topic/safety/clinical-decision-support>; 2018 Accessed 21.04.18.
3. Agency for Healthcare Research and Quality. Section 2—overview of CDS five rights. <https://healthit.ahrq.gov/ahrq-funded-projects/current-health-it-priorities/clinical-decision-support-cds/chapter-1-approaching-clinical-decision/section-2-overview-cds-five-rights>; Accessed 21.04.18.

Q 1.3: b. Meaningful Use

In 2009, the Health Information Technology for Economic and Clinical Health Act established objectives that providers must meet to demonstrate appropriate and meaningful use of their EHRs to receive an incentive payment. The goal was to show Centers for Medicare and Medicaid Services that providers are using their EHRs in ways that can affect patient care in positive ways. The program

was to be rolled out in three stages: Stage 1 focused on the capture of data and sharing, Stage 2 focused on advancing clinical processes, and Stage 3 focused on improving clinical outcomes for patients.

Suggested further reading

1. Centers for Medicare and Medicaid Services. An introduction to the Medicaid EHR incentive program for eligible professionals. <https://www.cms.gov/Regulations-and-Guidance/Legislation/EHRIncentive-Programs/Downloads/EHR_Medicaid_Guide_Remediated_2012.pdf>; Accessed 28.04.18.

Q 1.4: e. All of the above

Electronic health records (EHRs) can offer a number of advantages to help providers deliver better health care and improved coordinated care for patients. EHRs offer the ability to prescribe medications in a safer and reliable manner, enable improved care by ease of timely access to patient records, promote accurate and complete documentation, and improve efficiency and productivity by providing up-to-date information about a patient's health at that point of care, among many other advantages.

Suggested further reading

1. Office of the National Coordinator for Health Information Technology. What are the advantages of electronic health records? <https://www.healthit.gov/providers-professionals/faqs/what-are-advantages-electronic-health-records>; 2018 Accessed 23.04.18.

Q 1.5: a. Health Level 7

Health Level 7 (HL7) is one of the data exchange standards currently used to enable one health care institution to talk to another. HL7 provides a standard vehicle to share, exchange, and retrieve health information electronically. Multiple versions of HL7 exist; however, HL7 Version 2 is dominant in the United States and allows the exchange of patient admission/discharge/transfer information, laboratory orders, immunizations, and many other types of information. HL7 is used to facilitate data exchange among systems within an institution, as well as between institutions. For example, a laboratory information system may use HL7 to transfer data into a patient's clinical record. Many other standards have been developed for data exchange in the health care setting such as CDA, HL7 Version 3, and FHIR.

Digital Imaging and Communications in Medicine (DICOM) is an international standard for the exchange, storage, and communication of medical images and other related data. Hypertext Markup Language (HTML) is a standardized system that defines the structure of a webpage and its content. Current Procedural Terminology (CPT) is a coding system allowing physicians a uniform process for coding medical services that increases efficiency and accuracy among many other benefits. Cascading Style Sheets (CSS) helps describe how elements of HTML are displayed in a website or in other types of media. CSS can control how several webpages look all at once.

Suggested further reading

1. American Medical Association. CPT® purpose & mission. <https://www.ama-assn.org/practice-management/cpt-purpose-mission>; Accessed 07.08.18.

Q 1.6: d. Prescription Drug Monitoring Program

A prescription drug monitoring program (PDMP) contains information on all controlled substance prescriptions prescribed in a state. The database is electronic and allows the monitoring of dispensed prescriptions. A PDMP can offer information to providers and health authorities about prescriptions dispensed, and offer ease of use via an online portal or integration into an EHR, real time data retrieval about filled controlled substances, and universal use. Many states have mandated prescribers check the PDMP prior to each initiation of a controlled substance prescription.

Suggested further reading

1. Centers for Disease Control and Prevention. What states need to know about PDMPs. <https://www.cdc.gov/drugoverdose/pdmp/states.html>; 2017 Accessed 31.03.18.

Case 2 answers

Q 2.1: d. Both a and c

A data warehouse is a collection of data that has been extracted from a larger database or multiple other databases. The data warehouse allows the opportunity to do analytics on a portion of a database instead of the larger full set database. It is important to separate these portions of data from larger databases for analytic and reporting purposes because continued query of a single database could cause performance issues of the larger clinical systems. The warehousing of data (whenever the data are moved from the larger database to the data warehouse) usually occurs during times of reduced demand; however, depending on the urgency of the data need, periodic query during busier times would be more appropriate. This data separation allows quicker querying, reporting, and analysis of data.

Q 2.2: d. International Classification of Diseases (ICD)

The ICD is a standard that was introduced in the late 1970s to record inpatient procedures and diagnoses. Since October 2015, the US health care system has used the ICD-10 code set. Using these codes offers several benefits for patients and public health agencies. This expanded code set allows systematic research to be undertaken on the diseases. The ICD-10 codes can be used for sufficient reimbursement claims, distinguish risk and severity of disease, and provide more precise descriptions of the ailment. The Fast Health Interoperability Resources (FHIR) specification is a standard championed by HL7 to electronically exchange health care information. Logical Observation and Identifiers Names and Codes (LOINC) is a standard initiated in 1994 by the Regenstrief Institute. It is used to identify health measurements, observations, and documents. LOINC is most notable as a common language for laboratory results. RxNorm is a system that was created to help normalize the names for generic and brand name drugs. This system also allows interoperability between drug terminologies and pharmacy management systems. The Gold Standard Disease Databank (choice e) is simply a distractor with no appropriate meaning.

Suggested further reading

1. American Medical Association. ICD-10. <https://www.ama-assn.org/practice-management/icd-10>; Accessed 23.08.18.

Q 2.3: a. Discharge summary

Structured data can be entered into specific fields that have predefined purposes. The data can be forced to have a standardized format (e.g., a phone number field). Some examples of structured data would be vital signs, patient demographics, and laboratory results. Unstructured data cannot be organized as easily into these predetermined fields. Another way to think of unstructured data is to think of it as unorganized and potentially including a lot of text. Some examples of unstructured data in health care are clinical notes (this would include discharge summaries), free-text fields, and images. Other examples of unstructured data outside of the health care realm would be email messages and text messages.

Suggested further readings

1. Beaulieu-Jones BK. Machine learning for structured clinical data. <https://arxiv.org/abs/1707.06997v1>; 2017 Accessed 23.08.18.
2. HIMSS. FY16 HIE in practice task force. Blending structured and unstructured data to develop healthcare insights. <https://www.himss.org/library/blending-structured-and-unstructured-data-develop-healthcare-insights>; 2016 Accessed 23.08.18.

Q 2.4: d. Both a and c

The Digital Imaging and Communication in Medicine (DICOM) format provides a number of benefits to the medical community. DICOM allows the transmission, storage, process, and display of medical imaging information. The transition from film images to digital images has made the DICOM standard necessary. When using film, differences in exposure and processing will have little effect on the communication, display, and storage of these images; however, differences in computer coding can make it extremely difficult to transfer the document from one computer to another. The adaptability of the standard has allowed its adoption by a number of different specialties. DICOM is usually viewed as a set of standards rather than a single standalone standard. DICOM is far from the only standard currently used in health care. Some of the better known standards are Health Level 7 (HL7) and Logical Observation and Identifiers Names and Codes (LOINC). LOINC is a standard that was initiated in 1994 by the Regenstrief Institute. It is used to identify health measurements, observations, and documents. LOINC is most notable because it is a common language for laboratory results. HL7 Version 2 is a messaging standard that was developed by Health Level 7 and was initially released in 1987. HL7 Version 2 allows the exchange of health care data between systems. It is arguably the most widely implemented standard in the health care domain. The DICOM standard is used in the United States and many other countries worldwide.

Suggested further readings

1. Horii SC. Primer on computers and information technology. Part four: a nontechnical introduction to DICOM. *Radiographics*. 1997;17(5):1297-1309.
2. DICOM. *Home*. National Electrical Manufacturers Association. <https://www.dicomstandard.org/>; Accessed 23.08.18.
3. Pianykh OS. What is DICOM? In: *Digital Imaging and Communications in Medicine (DICOM)*. Berlin, Heidelberg: Springer.
4. Regenstrief. What LOINC is. <https://loinc.org/get-started/what-loinc-is/>; Accessed 08.08.18.
5. Health Level Seven International. HL7 messaging standard version 2.7. <http://www.hl7.org/implement/standards/product_brief.cfm?product_id=146>; Accessed 12.08.18.

Q 2.5: b. Improved coordinated care

EHRs have a number of benefits, including 88% of doctors reporting that their EHR produced a clinical benefit for their practice and 75% reporting that their EHR allowed them to deliver better patient care, according to a survey of doctors by the National Center for Health Statistics. However, many pain points continue to exist, including reductions in productivity, less time for face-to-face patient care, and increases in physician burnout. One survey in 2016 found that 84.5% of doctors in active practices used EHRs. Physicians who used EHRs reported feeling less satisfied and were also found to be at higher risk of burnout. Some studies have shown an increase in cognitive load and a decrease in productivity. EHRs are a great tool to augment the practice of providers; however, steps still need to be taken to continuously update and improve the end user's experience. EHRs are able to improve care by fostering improved coordination. According to the Office of the National Coordinator for Health Information Technology, "Electronic health record (EHR) systems can decrease the fragmentation of care by improving care coordination. EHRs have the potential to integrate and organize patient health information and facilitate its instant distribution among all authorized providers involved in a patient's care. For example, EHR alerts can be used to notify providers when a patient has been in the hospital, allowing them to proactively follow up with the patient."

Suggested further readings

1. Collier R. Electronic health records contributing to physician burnout. *Can Med Assoc J*. 2017;189(45):E1405-E1406.
2. Wolver S. EHR: pearls and pitfalls. Presented at Virginia ACP. <https://www.acponline.org/system/files/ documents/about_acp/chapters/va/15mtg/wolver.pdf>; March 7, 2015 Accessed 23.08.18.
3. The Office of the National Coordinator for Health Information Technology. Improve care coordination. <https://www.healthit.gov/topic/health-it-basics/improve-care-coordination>; 2017 Accessed 13.08.18.

Case 3 answers

Q 3.1: d. A clinical data registry is a record of the health status of a patient and the health care he or she has received over a period of time

A clinical data registry usually focuses on patients who share a common theme for needing health care. This is a place where providers and others can view patients who have received different treatments and what treatments are available for this disease process. The information can be used to assess health care professional outcomes, utilization of resources, among other topics. A center may choose not to participate in a specific disease clinical data registry for a number of reasons. It is not required for a center that treats a specific disease to have access to a clinical data registry; however, it is of benefit to the patient and provider. One large benefit of a clinical registry is the ability to query data for research. Health care professionals can send encrypted data about patients to the clinical data registry through a highly secure web portal or from their electronic health record. As data enter the clinical data registry, quality checks are performed to ensure the correctness and completeness of the data. If something is missing or outside of the expected range, registry staff contact the submitting health care professionals to ask them to review and verify the data.

Suggested further readings

1. Centers for Disease Control and Prevention. National Amyotrophic Lateral Sclerosis (ALS) Registry. <https://www.cdc.gov/als/Default.html>; 2018 Accessed 14.04.18.
2. National Quality Registry Network. What is a clinical data registry? <https://www.abms.org/media/1358/what-is-a-clinical-data-registry.pdf>; 2014 Accessed 14.04.18.

Q 3.2: e. All of the above

Technology in health care has improved the health and quality of life for patients all over the world. Telehealth services allow individuals in rural and underserved areas access to health care. Advances in IT have continued to make significant contributions through the increased use of EHRs. Mobile technologies allow individuals access to remote monitoring, test results, and information at their fingertips. Physicians and patients are more connected than ever.

Q 3.3: b. Clinical informatics

According to Oregon Health & Science University's definition, clinical informatics can be described as "informatics applied to health care or individual health settings. The application of informatics focused on specific health care disciplines usually includes the name of that discipline, such as nursing, dentistry, pathology, etc...." According to the American Medical Informatics Association, "Translational Bioinformatics is the development of storage, analytics, and interpretive methods to optimize the transformation of increasingly voluminous biomedical, and genomic data, into proactive, predictive, preventive, and participatory health." Also according to the American Medical Informatics Association, "Public Health Informatics is the application of informatics in areas of public health, including surveillance, prevention, preparedness, and health promotion." According to Oregon Health & Science University's definition, imaging informatics is "informatics with a focus on imaging, including the use of PACS system to store and retrieve images in health care settings."

Suggested further readings

1. Oregon Health and Science University. What is biomedical informatics? <http://www.ohsu.edu/xd/education/schools/school-of-medicine/departments/clinical-departments/dmice/about/what-is-biomedical-informatics.cfm>; Accessed 23.08.18.
2. American Medical Informatics Association. Translational bioinformatics. <https://www.amia.org/applications-informatics/translational-bioinformatics>; Accessed 23.08.18.
3. American Medical Informatics Association. Public health informatics. <https://www.amia.org/applications-informatics/public-health-informatics>; Accessed 23.08.18.

Case 4 answers

Q 4.1: e. All of the above

According to the Food and Drug Administration, a medical device is defined as "an instrument, apparatus, implement, machine, contrivance, implant, in vitro reagent, or other similar or related article, including a component part or accessory which is: recognized in the official National Formulary, or the United States Pharmacopoeia, or any supplement to them, intended for use in the diagnosis of disease or other conditions, or in the cure, mitigation, treatment, or prevention of disease, in man or other animals, or intended to affect the structure or any function of the body of man or other animals, and which does not achieve its primary intended purposes through chemical action within or on the body of man or other animals and which is not dependent upon being metabolized for the achievement of any of its primary intended purposes." All of the listed items are considered medical devices.

Suggested further readings

1. Food and Drug Administration. Products and medical procedures. <https://www.fda.gov/MedicalDevices/ProductsandMedicalProcedures/ucm2005078.htm>; 2018 Accessed 23.08.18.
2. Food and Drug Administration. Medical device overview. <https://www.fda.gov/ForIndustry/ImportProgram/ImportBasics/RegulatedProducts/ucm510630.htm>; 2017 Accessed 23.08.18.

Q 4.2: c. Class III

The Food and Drug Administration regulates devices by classifying them into three categories. The classification depends on the intended use of the device and the indications for use. Additionally, the classification is risk based. Class I includes devices with the lowest risk to patients and/or users, and Class III includes those with the highest risk. An example of a Class I device would be a set of examination gloves. An example of a Class II device would be a powered wheelchair, and an example of a Class III device would include a silicone gel-filled breast implant. As of August 2018, no class IV medical device exists, thus answer choice d is a distractor.

Suggested further readings

1. Food and Drug Administration. Classify your medical device. <https://www.fda.gov/MedicalDevices/DeviceRegulationandGuidance/Overview/ClassifyYourDevice/ucm2005371.htm>; 2018 Accessed 23.08.18.
2. Food and Drug Administration. Information sheet guidance for IRBs, clinical investigators, and sponsors—frequently asked questions about medical devices. <https://www.fda.gov/downloads/RegulatoryInformation/Guidances/UCM127067.pdf>; 2006 Accessed 31.03.18.

Q 4.3: d. Both a and c

According to the World Health Organization, telemedicine is "the delivery of health care services, where distance is a critical factor, by all health care professionals using information and communication technologies for the exchange of valid information for diagnosis, treatment and prevention of disease and injuries, research and evaluation, and for the continuing education of health care providers, all in the interests of advancing the health of individuals and their communities." Particularly in the United States, telemedicine allows several benefits to the patient, including enhanced access to care, improved patient satisfaction, and cost reduction. Telemedicine also has the potential to mitigate the national physician shortage. Not all private and public insurers pay for telemedicine visits; however, a large number will pay for them. Medicare does pay for telemedicine visits in certain circumstances such as a telehealth consultation in the emergency department on an initial inpatient consult. Medicaid covers at least some telehealth services; however, the coverage in each state varies. Many private insurers cover at least some telehealth services, and many insurers have expressed interest in expanding coverage of telehealth. Thirty-four states and Washington, DC, require that private insurers cover telehealth visits as they would any other visit.

Suggested further readings

1. American Telemedicine Association. Telemedicine benefits. <http://www.americantelemed.org/main/about/about-telemedicine/telemedicine-benefits>; Accessed 25.03.18.
2. Becker's Hospital Review. Telemedicine laws and developments: a state-by-state analysis. Becker's Health IT

and CIO Report. <https://www.beckershospitalreview. com/healthcare-information-technology/telemedicine-laws-and-developments-a-state-by-state-analysis.html>; 2014 Accessed 23.08.18.

3. World Health Organization. Telemedicine: opportunities and developments in member states. <http://www.who. int/goe/publications/goe_telemedicine_2010.pdf>; 2010 Accessed 28.04.18.

4. American Telemedicine Association. About telemedicine. <http://www.americantelemed.org/main/about/ telehealth-faqs->; Accessed 13.08.18.

Q 4.4: e. Health Insurance Portability and Accountability Act (HIPAA)

HIPAA, enacted in 1996, required the Department of Health and Human Services to create standards to protect the privacy and security of health information. The HIPAA Privacy Rule was published to shelter the privacy of individual's health information. The Security Rule created a set of standards for protecting health information that is transferred or retained in an electronic form.

Suggested further reading

1. Department of Health and Human Services. Summary of the HIPAA security rule. <https://www.hhs.gov/hipaa/ for-professionals/security/laws-regulations/index.html>; 2013 Accessed 26.03.18.

Q 4.5: e. All of the above

Predictive analytics can be used to make predictions about future events. Many techniques are used with current and historical data to help model and predict these future events such as machine learning, data mining, advanced analytics, and predictive modeling. Predictive analytics uses a potential number of techniques and variables that are weighted appropriately by the model designer to conclude relationships that will, in the end, produce a prediction. Machine learning is a technique to analyze data that teaches computers and other devices to learn information from the data given to it. Machine learning uses algorithms to learn the data and, as more data and examples are supplied, the computer is able to improve its performance. Data mining is a data analytic technique to explore large amounts of data in search of relationships between variables. Predictive models analyze trends in past data in an attempt to predict future relationships and trends. A number of models and techniques are typically used to help create and validate the model to predict an outcome.

Case 5 answers

Q 5.1: a. Increased ability to reach underserved populations

Mobile Health (mHealth) is defined by the World Health Organization as the "medical and public health practice supported by mobile devices, such as mobile phones, patient monitoring devices, personal digital assistances, and other wireless devices." In a 2014 study by S. Akter et al. mHealth offered an unprecedented opportunity to serve underserved populations. Evidence is continuing to become apparent that mHealth has already transformed the delivery of some types of health care in poor settings. Some of the other benefits of mHealth include convenience, education, and the encouragement of a healthy lifestyle. A *JAMA* study published in 2016 showed that over 148,000 units of mHealth applications were sold to help estimate blood pressure. The technique used to measure the blood pressure in the application was to place the top edge of the smartphone on the left side of a user's chest while the user also placed his or her index finger over the smartphone's camera. The study showed that approximately 77.5% of individuals with hypertensive blood pressure levels will be falsely reassured that their blood pressure was in a nonhypertensive range. The FDA regulates certain mobile applications, but not all.

Suggested further readings

1. Akter S, Ray P. mHealth—an ultimate platform to serve the unserved. *Yearb Med Inform*. 2010:94-100.

2. Anglada-Martinez H, Riu-Viladoms G, Martin-Conde M, Rovira-Illamola M, Sotoca-Momblona JM, Codina-Jane C. Does mHealth increase adherence to medication? Results of a systematic review. *Int J Clin Pract*. 2015; 69(1):9-32.

3. Plante TB, Urrea B, MacFarlane ZT, et al. Validation of the instant blood pressure smartphone app. *JAMA Intern Med*. 2016;176(5):700-702.

4. Food and Drug Administration. Examples of MMAs the FDA Regulates. <https://www.fda.gov/MedicalDevices/ DigitalHealth/MobileMedicalApplications/ucm368743. htm>; 2015 Accessed 13.08.18.

5. Food and Drug Administration. Mobile medical applications. <https://www.fda.gov/medicaldevices/ digitalhealth/mobilemedicalapplications/default.htm>; 2018 Accessed 13.08.18.

Q 5.2: d. Indexed HIE model

The indexed HIE model is not an example of an HIE architecture. Direct HIE is an example of an HIE architecture. One of the best ways to think about the direct model is to think of it as secure emailing. Members of a health care team are sending information about a patient from one place to another. It is easy and secure; however, this is not the answer for large-scale exchanges of data. In the centralized model, the patient's medical data are collected from authorized providers periodically and stored in a central repository. Requests from permitted providers can query this central database and view the patient's medical data. The decentralized model allows the provider to maintain control and ownership over the patient's medical data. In this model, there is no central repository, instead the data are collected from that provider by those authorized to access the record. Fig. 3.1 displays the common HIE technical architecture models.

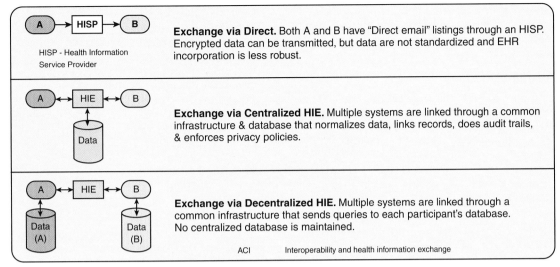

Exchange via Direct. Both A and B have "Direct email" listings through an HISP. Encrypted data can be transmitted, but data are not standardized and EHR incorporation is less robust.

HISP - Health Information Service Provider

Exchange via Centralized HIE. Multiple systems are linked through a common infrastructure & database that normalizes data, links records, does audit trails, & enforces privacy policies.

Data

Exchange via Decentralized HIE. Multiple systems are linked through a common infrastructure that sends queries to each participant's database. No centralized database is maintained.

Data (A)   Data (B)

ACI   Interoperability and health information exchange

Fig. 3.1 HIMSS. Common HIE technical architecture models.

Q 5.3: e. Both c and d

According to the US Department of Health and Human Services, "Encryption is a method of converting an original message of regular text into encoded text. The text is encrypted by means of an algorithm (type of formula). If information is encrypted, there would be a low probability that anyone other than the receiving party who has the key to the code or access to another confidential process would be able to decrypt (translate) the text and convert it into plain, comprehensible text." Encryption (choice d) is a method used to preserve the patient's data integrity and confidentiality. Authentication (choice c) is needed when a user is producing proof of his or her identity to a computer server.

Suggested further readings

1. Hackworth R. Data encryption. *Compute Bull.* 1995;37(6):12-13.
2. Department of Health and Human Services. What is encryption? <https://www.hhs.gov/hipaa/for-professionals/faq/2021/what-is-encryption/index.html>; 2013 Accessed 14.04.18.

Q 5.4: a. Metadata

The American Health Information Management Association defines metadata as "descriptive data that characterize other data to create a clearer understanding of their meaning and to achieve greater reliability and quality of information." An example of metadata is the data created about a patient's record whenever it is accessed, created, or changed. Another example of metadata is the time stamp whenever documents or images are uploaded to a patient's chart.

Suggested further reading

1. Haugen MB, Herrin B, Slivochka S, Tolley LM, Warner D, Washington L. Rules for handling and maintaining metadata in the EHR. *J AHIMA.* 2013;84(5):50-54.

Q 5.5: e. All of the above

Computerized provider order entry (CPOE) allows a number of advantages over traditional ordering via a paper system. Some advantages include avoiding problems associated with handwriting legibility and similar names of medications ordered. CPOE also allows for clinical decision support integration to check potential drug interactions. CPOE also has many other uses including e-prescribing transmission to pharmacies, rapid laboratory studies and radiological studies, among many other benefits. The electronic integration allows the ability to also recommend alternative tests that may be safer or lower cost to the patient at the time of order entry.

Suggested further reading

1. Agency for Healthcare Research and Quality. Computerized provider order entry. <https://psnet.ahrq.gov/primers/primer/6/computerized-provider-order-entry>; 2018 Accessed 25.04.18.

Q 5.6: a. Patient portal

According to the Office of the National Coordinator for Health Information Technology, a patient portal is "a secure online website that gives patients convenient, 24-hour access to personal health information from anywhere with an Internet connection." Patients are able to log in to their account and view medications, immunizations, lab results, and a number of other health care–related items.

In 2009, the Health Information Technology for Economic and Clinical Health Act established objectives that providers must meet to demonstrate appropriate and meaningful use of their EHRs to receive an incentive payment. The goal was to show Centers for Medicare and Medicaid that providers are using their EHRs in ways that can affect patient care in positive ways. The Meaningful Use program was to be rolled out in three stages: Stage 1 focused on the capture of data and sharing, Stage 2 focused on advancing clinical processes, and Stage 3 focused on improving clinical outcomes for patients.

Suggested further readings

1. Centers for Medicare and Medicaid Services. Stage 2 overview tipsheet. <https://www.cms.gov/Regulations-and-Guidance/Legislation/EHRIncentivePrograms/Downloads/Stage2Overview_Tipsheet.pdf>; 2012 Accessed 28.04.18.

2. Office of the National Coordinator for Health Information Technology. What is a patient portal? <https://www.healthit.gov/faq/what-patient-portal>; 2017 Accessed 28.04.18.

3. Centers for Medicare and Medicaid Services. An introduction to the Medicaid EHR incentive program for eligible professionals. <https://www.cms.gov/Regulations-and-Guidance/Legislation/EHRIncentivePrograms/Downloads/EHR_Medicaid_Guide_Remediated_2012.pdf>; Accessed 28.04.18.

4

Socioecologic Determinants of Health

Eliana V. Hempel, MD

Cases and questions

Case 1

Mrs. Gurung, a 31-year-old G1-P0 Bhutanese woman who is approximately 30 weeks pregnant, presents to the women's health clinic for initial evaluation. She immigrated to the United States from a Nepali refugee camp 2 months ago. She has had no prenatal care to date. She only speaks Nepali, but is accompanied by her husband, who speaks a little bit of English. An interpreter phone is used to conduct most of the interview. She complains of severe, diffuse body pain. Her physical examination is unremarkable, and initial laboratory assessment reveals no underlying etiology for her pain. She does not present for her initial follow-up appointment.

Q 1.1: In addition to issues related to her provider's cultural competency, what other social determinants of health may be contributing to Mrs. Gurung's failure to follow up?
a. Lack of health insurance
b. Lack of financial resources
c. Transportation
d. All of the above

Case 2

Mrs. Gurung also does not attend subsequent follow-up appointments. She then presents to the emergency department at approximately 39 weeks' gestation with severe abdominal pain. Her assessment shows that she is in active labor. Nepali custom dictates that Mr. Gurung not be present in the delivery room. Mrs. Gurung does well until she is fully dilated, and it is time for her to push. No interpreters are available, and she cannot understand what to do.

Q 2.1: Which of the following represents culturally competent behavior on the part of the provider?
a. Recruitment of a female family member or friend to assist with interpretation during delivery
b. Insistence that Mr. Gurung attend the delivery and assist with interpretation
c. Enlistment of a Nepali administrative staff member for interpretation during delivery
d. Utilization of a professional Nepali interpreter during the delivery

Q 2.2: Will Mrs. Gurung's child be impacted by the social determinants of health to which she was exposed at birth?
a. Yes, children born to parents who live in poverty and mothers who have poor nutritional status during pregnancy are more likely to have poor health outcomes as adults
b. Yes, but only if these social determinants of health persist during childhood
c. No, though low socioeconomic status has been linked to complications during pregnancy, it has not been linked to long-term poor health outcomes for the child
d. No, because correlation does not equal causality

Case 3

Mr. Peterson is a 47-year-old Caucasian male with diabetes and hypertension. He presents to the outpatient clinic for follow-up. During his last visit, his hemoglobin A1c was noted to be 8.1% and his blood pressure was 153/92 mmHg. The physician initiated metformin and lisinopril and provided Mr. Peterson with an informational packet about diabetes. He was also asked to record his blood sugars and blood pressures and bring in a log of these values to his next visit. On presentation today, his repeat blood work shows a hemoglobin A1c of 8.4%. His blood pressure is 157/94 mmHg.

He has not completed a blood sugar or blood pressure log. He is asked to write down his recent blood sugars from memory, and he communicates that he is unable to do so because he does not know how to read or write.

Q 3.1: In patients like Mr. Peterson, which of the following educational interventions has been most strongly linked to improved health outcomes over time?

a. Community health education talks regarding chronic diseases
b. Adult literacy programs
c. Early and sustained basic and generalized educational experiences
d. Health education in the public school setting

Q 3.2: Which of the following statements is FALSE regarding assessment of health literacy by medical professionals?

a. The most commonly used health literacy assessment tools are the Rapid Assessment of Adult Literacy in Medicine (REALM) and the Test of Functional Health Literacy in Adults (TOFHLA)
b. The focus of most health literacy assessment tools is print literacy
c. Patients who always take paperwork home to complete may have problems with literacy and should be screened
d. Educational level attained correlates moderately well with health literacy

Case 4

You explain the complications of diabetes to Mr. Peterson. He reports that he now understands why it is important to take his medications. He also expresses an interest in trying to change his diet, to help with his blood sugar control.

Q 4.1: Successful dietary changes would represent which of the following outcomes?

a. Health promotion actions
b. Health promotion outcomes
c. Intermediate health outcomes
d. Health and social outcomes

Q 4.2: Which of the following factors is most significantly linked to premature death?

a. Genetics
b. Social and environmental factors
c. Individual behaviors
d. Health care

Case 5

Mr. Rivera, an obese 55-year-old, uninsured, Hispanic male presents to the emergency department after 4 hours of crushing, substernal chest pain. He reports that he has no known past medical history and is a nonsmoker. He describes recent increased stress because, though he has an associate degree, he recently lost his job and has been unable to find new employment. His vital signs are significant for a blood pressure of 165/95 mmHg. A basic metabolic panel is notable for a blood sugar of 180 mg/dL. An electrocardiogram shows no signs of acute ischemia or left ventricular hypertrophy. Serial troponins are negative. He is discharged from the emergency

department with the phone number for the nearest free clinic to establish care and obtain a stress test.

Q 5.1: Which of the following personal characteristics makes Mr. Rivera more likely to re-present to the emergency department?

a. Race
b. Educational status
c. Health status
d. Gender

Q 5.2: Which of the following statements is TRUE?

a. Mr. Rivera is more likely to be underweight due to his low income, compared to similar patients with higher incomes
b. Mr. Rivera is more likely to be obese than his wife
c. Mr. Rivera's lack of insurance makes it more likely that he will not seek out further medical care
d. All of the above statements are true

Case 6

Mr. Rivera returns to the emergency department 1 year later with recurrent, severe chest pain. He is found to have an ST-elevation myocardial infarction and is urgently taken to the cardiac catheterization laboratory. He is found to have severe, three-vessel disease and is admitted for coronary artery bypass surgery.

Q 6.1: If implemented at the time of his initial emergency department visit, which of the following interventions would most likely have prevented his current complication of uncontrolled hypertension?

a. A patient education pamphlet on hypertension
b. A more extensive workup such as measurement of hemoglobin A1c and lipid profile during his initial emergency department stay
c. A scheduled appointment with a local clinic prior to discharge from the emergency department
d. Enrollment in a postemergency case management program

Q 6.2: On further questioning regarding his history, Mr. Rivera reports that, after his initial emergency department visit, he was subsequently seen in two other local emergency departments for symptoms related to high blood pressure. He states that, if someone had asked him, he would have explained why he was having difficulty following up with his primary care provider. Which of the following is LEAST likely to address provider-related barriers to addressing social determinants of health in the clinical setting?

a. Transitioning from a volume-based, fee-for-service payment system to a value-based payment system
b. Educating providers to not only screen for social determinants that may be affecting a patient's health but also to provide resources to address identified needs
c. Utilizing multidisciplinary care teams to provide comprehensive care
d. Promoting the move toward shift work and hospitalist care versus ambulatory care practice models

Case 7

Ms. Parker is a 44-year-old woman with peripheral neuropathy who presents to the emergency department for foot pain.

She denies any recent history of trauma but does report limited sensation in her feet. On exam, she is disheveled and appears older than her stated age. She is hemodynamically stable and, on evaluation of her foot, noted to have a wound on her left heel. The wound is shallow but without purulent discharge. There is mild tenderness to palpation but no surrounding erythema or warmth to palpation. Inflammatory markers are within normal limits, and she has no leukocytosis. Ms. Parker is given instructions on proper wound care and referred to her primary care physician for further follow-up.

Q 7.1: When considering management of a chronic appearing wound, what social factors should be assessed?
a. Ability to keep the wound clean
b. Ability to perform dressing changes
c. Adequate social support
d. All of the above

Case 8

Ms. Parker returns to the emergency department 3 weeks later with worsening pain. She is now hypotensive and tachycardic. Her foot wound is bandaged, but the bandage is dirty. Her wound is draining purulent discharge, and the surrounding skin is more erythematous and warm to the touch. She is admitted for a suspected skin and soft tissue infection with plans to receive intravenous (IV) antibiotics. She reports to the admitting team that she was recently evicted from her home. She was not able to purchase the prescribed dressing supplies and has not had consistent access to a bathroom.

Q 8.1: Which of the following statements is TRUE regarding housing instability in the United States?
a. The proportion of households that spends more than 50% of income on housing is 7%
b. The proportion of households that spends more than 30% of income on housing is 15%
c. Residential crowding is associated with physical ailments, but not psychologic distress
d. Moving three or more times in a year, or multiple moves, is associated with negative health outcomes in children
e. Of the homeless youth in America, 25% identify as lesbian, gay, bisexual, or transgender

Case 9

You subsequently see another patient, Mrs. Fletcher. She is the same age as Ms. Parker, has a very similar history, and also presents with foot pain due to a foot ulcer. Mrs. Fletcher developed her ulcer due to poor footwear. She is a high school teacher and is married to an accountant. You treat Mrs. Fletcher the same way you treated Ms. Parker. Mrs. Fletcher's ulcer improves much more quickly, and she suffers no complications.

Q 9.1: In the setting of similar medical histories and treatment plans, Mrs. Fletcher's difference in clinical course is an example of which of the following?
a. Social justice
b. Social gradient

c. Social structures
d. Social norms

Case 10

Mr. Harris is a 61-year-old male, with a 30 pack-years smoking history, who presents to the emergency department in January for shortness of breath. Though he was previously following up with a physician at the local free clinic, he has not followed up with her for the past 2 years. He reports that this is because he "doesn't like doctors." On initial examination, he is found to have hypoxemia (low oxygen saturations) and diffuse wheezes in all lung fields. He is diagnosed with a chronic obstructive pulmonary disease (COPD) exacerbation and admitted to the hospital. On further questioning, the physician finds out that he lives in an apartment building with a known mold problem. He also recently lost his job as a truck driver. Due to increased stress, he has since gone from smoking 1 pack/day to 2 packs/day.

Q 10.1: Which of the following is LEAST likely to have contributed to his recent admissions?
a. Built environment
b. Access to health care
c. Annual income
d. Occupation

Q 10.2: Differences in outcomes in patients with low socioeconomic status compared to patients with high socioeconomic status are an example of which of the following?
a. Health inequality
b. Health care disparity
c. Determinants of health
d. Health equity

Q 10.3: Taking into consideration the social determinants of health that are affecting Mr. Harris's COPD, which of the following community-based interventions is most likely to affect long-term outcomes related to his COPD?
a. Community-based smoking cessation classes
b. Health education classes in local elementary schools that focus on the dangers of tobacco use
c. Community legal services aimed to compel apartment management to address the mold problem in his apartment building
d. Low-cost medication assistance program that would help him obtain his medications

Case 11

Mr. Smith is an 82-year-old African American male with a past medical history of end-stage heart failure. He is a veteran of the US Army. He previously worked in construction but has been retired for many years. Mr. Smith currently lives alone in an urban setting, is divorced, and has two daughters. He is estranged from one of his daughters, but his younger daughter, Susan, has been involved in his care. She accompanies him to today's visit. He presents to his primary care provider's office for follow-up of his worsening heart failure symptoms. He reports that he has gained 5 pounds in the past week and feels dyspneic with minimal exertion. On exam, he is mildly tachycardic, his oxygen saturation is 90% on room air, and he has rales in the bases of his lungs bilaterally. Because of his symptom of dyspnea, he can barely leave the house. Due to poor eyesight, he no longer drives. However, he is still able to perform sedentary activities such as managing his finances. He fills his medications regularly and can describe how to take them appropriately. If Susan is not able to bring him meals, he typically gets his meals from the corner delicatessen. She expresses concern because she works three jobs and is unable to provide as much assistance with Mr. Smith's care as she would like. She inquires about other services that Mr. Smith may qualify for.

Q 11.1: Based on Mr. Smith's history, which of the following is LEAST likely to be contributing to his acute heart failure exacerbation?
a. Elder abuse
b. Social isolation
c. Access to low-sodium foods
d. Depression

Q 11.2: Which of the following social needs is most commonly unmet in older adults?
a. Financial security
b. Social connectedness
c. Adequate transportation
d. Food security

Q 11.3: In response to Susan's request for more resources, you refer Mr. Smith to the Area Agency on Aging (AAA). All of the following are TRUE about AAAs, EXCEPT:
a. AAAs receive federal funding through the Older Americans Act
b. AAAs are managed at the local level, to respond to the specific needs of the communities they serve
c. AAAs only serve Americans over the age of 60 years
d. The core services offered by all AAAs include elder rights, caregivers, nutrition, health and wellness, and supportive services

Case 12

You treat Mr. Smith for an acute heart failure exacerbation with increased diuretic dose and close monitoring. He improves to his baseline status. The Area Agency on Aging provides him with a meal delivery service and transportation assistance. Unfortunately, he is unable to afford the cost of home services. Two months later, he experiences another heart failure exacerbation, this time necessitating hospitalization. Susan is very worried that he can no longer care for himself at home. However, Mr. Smith is adamant about remaining at home for as long as possible.

Q 12.1: What services might you offer him, to try to manage his heart failure and keep him at home?
a. Home nursing services through the Programs for All-Inclusive Care for the Elderly (PACE)
b. Telemanagement of his heart failure
c. Veterans Affairs home-based primary care program
d. All of the above

Case 13

Cara is a 13-year-old girl with a past medical history of previously well-controlled type 1 diabetes mellitus. She presents to her pediatrician for follow-up after three inpatient admissions for diabetic ketoacidosis in the past 6 months. During her most recent hospitalization, her hemoglobin A1c was found to be 10%. Her discharge summary shows that her insulin regimen has been increased during each hospitalization, yet she keeps presenting with similar symptoms. She has gained 10 pounds in the past few months, and her body mass index now falls in the overweight range. During her visit, her pediatrician asks about social factors that may be contributing to the recent changes in the control of her diabetes. Her mother tearfully reports that, since taking a lower paying job, she has been having trouble making ends meet. Sometimes she decides between food for the family and Cara's medications. Though Cara's mom is aware of nutrition recommendations for diabetes, she is now having to rely on less expensive, highly processed, and carbohydrate-heavy foods.

Q 13.1: Which of the following statements regarding food insecurity is TRUE?
a. Urban food deserts are defined by lack of supermarket access within 0.25 mile of home
b. Greater access to supermarkets has not been linked to rates of overweight or obese individuals
c. Rates of food insecurity have been rising since 2009
d. Of children who are food insecure, 20% come from families that do not qualify for federal nutrition assistance programs

Q 13.2: You discuss several resources with Cara and her mother. You also ask them to keep a food diary, to get a better sense of what Cara is regularly eating. You explain to Cara and her mother that childhood obesity is linked to which of the following long-term complications?
a. Development of heart disease as an adult
b. Development of lung cancer as an adult
c. Development of tobacco dependence in adulthood
d. Development of anorexia nervosa in childhood

Q 13.3: Which of the following questions has been shown to be sensitive in screening for food insecurity?
a. In the last 12 months, how often have you been worried that food would run out before you got money to buy more?
b. In the last 12 months, how often have you had difficulty making ends meet at the end of the month?
c. In the last 24 hours, what have you eaten?
d. In the last month, how often have you gone grocery shopping?

Q 13.4: When screening for social determinants of health, which of the following strategies may help to avoid unintended consequences?
a. The use of risk-stratification tools to prompt automatic referrals
b. The use of sociodemographic factors to target screening
c. A focus on strengthening assets
d. All of the above

Answers

Case 1 answers

Q 1.1: d. All of the above

The term *social determinants of health* is defined in multiple ways. The Kaiser Family Foundation defines social determinants of health as "the structural determinants and conditions in which people are born, grow, live, work, and age." These social factors result in nearly one-third of US deaths annually. The determinants of health are further characterized in the Fig. 4.1. Mrs. Gurung is likely affected by multiple social determinants of health that are impacting the receipt of high-quality care. She may not have health insurance, financial resources, or access to transportation. Additionally, language barriers and other factors may also be contributing to her failure to follow up. A careful social history and a culturally sensitive approach may help mitigate some of these factors, to ensure improved patient care.

Case 2 answers

Q 2.1: d. Utilization of a professional Nepali interpreter during the delivery

Well-established data suggest that minority groups have higher rates of chronic diseases. Multiple factors likely contribute to this disparity. Cultural competency is defined as "a set of congruent behaviors, attitudes, and policies that come together in a system, agency, or amongst professionals, and enables that system, agency, or those professionals to work effectively in cross-cultural situations." Another definition of cultural competency is "the acknowledgement and incorporation—at all levels—of the importance of culture, assessment of cross-cultural relations, vigilance toward dynamics that result from cultural differences, expansion of cultural knowledge, and adaptation of services to meet culturally unique needs."

Additionally, more than 8% of Americans report limited English proficiency. Unfortunately, access to medical interpretation in health care delivery systems is not uniform or common. Furthermore, the majority of US teaching hospitals do not provide training in the use of medical interpreters. This significantly impacts patients as language barriers are linked to decreased patient satisfaction. In contrast, in one study, the use of professional interpreters, instead of ad hoc interpreters, resulted in increased patient comprehension, improved clinical outcomes, and improved patient satisfaction. Though both providers and interpreters rate in-person interpretation more highly than other modalities, patient satisfaction is unchanged between in-person, video, and telephonic interpretation.

Q 2.2: a. Yes, children born to parents who live in poverty and mothers who have poor nutritional status during pregnancy are more likely to have poor health outcomes as adults

Low socioeconomic status during pregnancy has been linked to long-term outcomes for offspring during both childhood and adulthood. Particularly, poor prenatal care and poor nutrition have strong associations with poor outcomes. In addition, children with low socioeconomic status seem to be more severely affected by the illnesses they develop. Low socioeconomic status continues to affect health if experienced during childhood and adolescence. However, exposures in utero can have significant impact, even if socioeconomic status improves during childhood. This highlights the importance of addressing social determinants of health in pregnant women and during childhood.

Economic Stability	Neighborhood and Physical Environment	Education	Food	Community and Social Context	Health Care System
Employment	Housing	Literacy	Hunger	Social integration	Health coverage
Income	Transportaion	Language	Access to healthy options	Support systems	Provider availability
Expenses	Safety	Early childhood education		Community engagement	Provider linguistic and cultural competency
Debt	Parks	Vocational Training		Discrimination	Quality of care
Medical bills	Playgrounds	Higher Education			
Support	Walkability				
	Zip code/geography				

Health Outcomes
Mortality, Morbidity, Life Expectancy, Health Care Expenditures, Health Status, Functional Limitations

Fig. 4.1 Social determinants of health. (From Henry J Kaiser Family Foundation. https://www.kff.org/disparities-policy/issue-brief/beyond-health-care-the-role-of-social-determinants-in-promoting-health-and-health-equity. Published November 4, 2015.)

Suggested further readings

1. Heiman H, Artiga S. *Beyond health care: the role of social determinants in promoting health and health equity.* Henry J Kaiser Family Foundation. <https://www.kff.org/disparities-policy/issue-brief/beyond-health-care-the-role-of-social-determinants-in-promoting-health-and-health-equity>; 2015 Accessed 01.03.18.
2. Flores G. Language barriers to health care in the United States. *N Engl J Med.* 2006;355:229-231.
3. Healthypeople.gov. Maternal, infant, and child health. <https://www.healthypeople.gov/2020/topics-objectives/topic/maternal-infant-and-child-health>; Accessed 03.03.18.

Case 3 answers

Q 3.1: c. Early and sustained basic and generalized educational experiences

Educational level is associated with overall health. Even though many communities use population health-based educational interventions to address community-specific health needs, generalized education starting at an early age has been most strongly linked to improved health outcomes. Low literacy is associated with a range of poor health outcomes. This is an international issue. The World Health Organization notes that literacy is a predictor of inequities across the world.

The US Department of Health and Human Services defines health literacy as "the degree to which individuals have the capacity to obtain, process, and understand basic health information and services needed to make appropriate decisions."

Health literacy includes the following skills:

- Ability to read and understand text and interpret information in documents
- Ability to use quantitative information for tasks
- Ability to speak and listen effectively

Q 3.2: d. Educational level attained correlates moderately well with health literacy

The most commonly used tools to assess health literacy are the Rapid Estimate of Adult Literacy in Medicine (REALM) and the Test of Functional Health Literacy in Adults (TOFHLA). REALM mainly assesses vocabulary, and TOFHLA measures reading fluency; however, these tools focus on only certain aspects that contribute to overall health literacy. Other screening tools exist, and researchers and clinicians alike have made recommendations for the development of tools that are simultaneously more comprehensive and easy to administer. Though clinicians often use "level of education achieved" as a measure of literacy, it does not correlate well with literacy or health literacy. For example, a Medicare managed care enrollee survey showed that up to 27% of high school graduates had inadequate or marginal health literacy. Signs that a patient is struggling with literacy-related issues and should be screened further include:

- Incorrectly or inaccurately completing paperwork
- Always taking paperwork home for completion
- Always bringing a friend or family member to the visit to help with completion of paperwork
- Giving excuses for why paperwork cannot be completed in the office, such as lack of eyeglasses

Case 4 answers

Q 4.1: c. Intermediate health outcomes

Lifestyle changes represent intermediate health outcomes. These intermediate outcomes will ultimately impact health and social outcomes. Long-term outcomes include health and social outcomes, which can include morbidity and mortality and quality of life. Health promotion outcomes are the immediate results of health promotion–related interventions. When developing health education–related interventions, it is important to take into consideration the circumstances of the community. If the population does not have the means or resources to act on the education they receive, it will not be as effective. Fig. 4.2 provides further descriptions and examples of these outcomes.

Q 4.2: c. Individual behaviors

In the United States, behavioral factors contribute to 40% of premature deaths. The two behaviors that are most associated with premature death are obesity/physical inactivity and smoking. However, as seen in Fig. 4.3, social and environmental factors also play a substantial role. Though genetic factors play a role in premature death, modification of genetic factors will require significant scientific advancement. Therefore, physicians who address social and environmental factors, as well as an individual's behaviors, will create the largest impact on preventable causes of death.

Suggested further readings

1. Schroeder S. We can do better—improving the health of the American people. *N Engl J Med.* 2007;257:1221-1228.
2. Berkman ND, Sheridan SL, Donahue KE, Halpern DJ, Crotty K. Low health literacy and health outcomes: an updated systematic review. *Ann Intern Med.* 2011;155(2):97-107.
3. Baker DW. The meaning and the measure of health literacy. *J Gen Intern Med.* 2006;21(8):878-883.

Case 5 answers

Q 5.1: b. Educational status

Many social factors play a role in patients' usual source of care. Usual source of care is the provider(s) identified by patients as the place they would go if ill or requiring health-related advice. The following factors are noted to be associated with increased utilization of the emergency department:

- Female sex
- Non-Hispanic black race
- Low household income
- Less than high school degree education level
- Poorer baseline health status
- Age older than 65 years

Lack of insurance has been debated as a possible source of increased emergency department utilization. Some studies have shown increased utilization in uninsured patients,

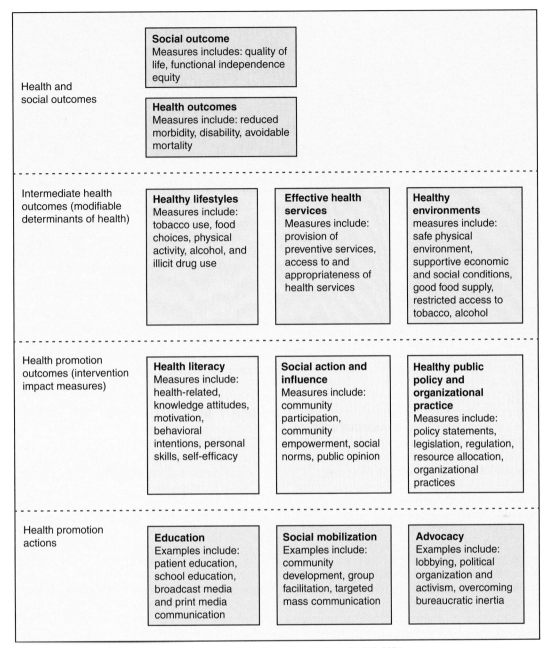

Fig. 4.2 Outcome model for health promotion. (From *Health Promot Int*. 2006; 15(3): 259-267.).

while others show no difference in utilization between insured and uninsured patients. In patients who identify a primary care provider as their usual source of care, emergency department utilization rates are still significant. Barriers to timely care contribute to frequent utilization of the emergency department, even in insured populations. Patient-reported barriers to timely care that are associated with higher emergency department utilization are:

- Inability to get through to their primary care office via phone
- Inability to obtain an appointment soon enough
- Prolonged wait times in the provider's office
- Inability to present to the provider's office during open office hours
- Lack of transportation

Q 5.2: c. Mr. Rivera's lack of insurance makes it more likely that he will not seek out further medical care

Obesity is more prevalent in lower income individuals. The rate of obesity in adults is highest (42.6%) in the group that makes 100% to 199% of the federal poverty line; the prevalence decreases (29.7%) in the group that makes 400% to 499% of the federal poverty line. White, black, and Hispanic women all tend to be more obese than their male counterparts. The greatest discrepancy is between non-Hispanic black women and men. More than double the percentage of patients without insurance postponed care or did not seek care due to cost, and reported having no usual source of care, compared to individuals with public or private insurance.

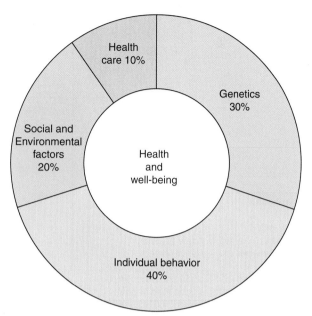

Fig. 4.3 Impact of different factors on risk of premature death. (Figure created and reprinted with permission of the Henry J Kaiser Family Foundation. Data source: Schroeder S. We can do better – improving the health of the American people. *N Engl J Med.* 2007; 257: 1221-1228.)

Case 6 answers

Q 6.1: d. Enrollment in a postemergency case management program

It is important to help patients shift from a model of seeking care only when ill, to seeking care proactively and continuously, with the aim of preventing illness. However, many patients experience innumerable barriers to continuous primary care. In patients without a primary care provider who are given a scheduled appointment prior to discharge from the emergency department, only about 50% attend these visits. In a systematic review focused on the efficacy of case management interventions after emergency department visits, most studies showed a reduction in the number of emergency department visits in patients who actively engaged with case management programs. Some studies also suggested that case management interventions result in more frequent follow-up with primary care providers. While increased education on his disease process and identification of additional comorbidities might have provided benefit, interventions geared toward increasing this patient's access to long-term, preventive care would be most likely to have had an impact on his progressive coronary artery disease.

Q 6.2: d. Promoting the move toward shift work and hospitalist care versus ambulatory care practice models

Mr. Rivera sought care in multiple settings for similar issues prior to his current hospitalization for advanced coronary artery disease. Likely, silos of care and lack of integration of the electronic health record contributed to his morbidity. Providers have identified multiple barriers to addressing social determinants of health, primarily lack of time and knowledge. Moving toward a value-based system that rewards providers for improvement in patients' overall health, rather than for the sheer number of patients seen, will help mitigate some of the

time-related barriers. Increasing provider comfort with identifying and addressing social determinants of health will also likely be effective in improving patient care. Developing a care system that incorporates a multidisciplinary team will provide the infrastructure required to successfully address patient needs. Furthering silos of care and requiring providers to assist patients in maneuvering the health system in settings in which they have never practiced may contribute to poor transitions of care.

Suggested further readings

1. Kamal R, Cox C, Blumenkranz E. *What do we know about social determinants of health in the U.S. and comparable countries?* Peterson-Kaiser Health System Tracker. <https://www.healthsystemtracker.org/chart-collection/know-social-determinants-health-u-s-comparable-countries/#item-start>; 2017 Accessed 14.04.18.
2. Naderi S, Barnett B, Hoffman RS, et al. Factors associated with failure to follow-up at a medical clinic after an ED visit. *Am J Emerg Med.* 2012;30(2):347-351.
3. Kumar GS, Klein R. Effectiveness of case management strategies in reducing emergency department visits in frequent user patient populations: a systematic review. *J Emerg Med.* 2013;44(3):717-729.

Case 7 answers

Q 7.1: d. All of the above

When managing chronic wounds, as with many chronic conditions, a clear understanding of patients' social history can prove critical. Particularly, patients' social capital can strongly influence their ability to manage their own health. Social capital is defined as "the benefits that accrue to individuals through their participation in cohesive groups or social networks." These benefits come in the form of social relationships that can be used to support the individual in times of need and to provide access to group resources. Unfortunately, patients are not often forthcoming about aspects of their social history that may cause them embarrassment or shame. Therefore, it is not only important to ask about patients' social situation but also to do so in a sensitive manner.

Case 8 answers

Q 8.1: d. Moving three or more times in a year, or multiple moves, is associated with negative health outcomes in children

Housing quality is defined by Healthypeople.gov as "the physical condition of a person's home as well as the quality of the social and physical environment in which the home is located." Housing instability may refer to difficulty paying for housing, spending most of one's income on housing, moving frequently, or staying with relatives. The proportion of households that spend a significant proportion of income on housing is substantial. Approximately 35% spend more than 30% on housing, while 15% spend more than 50% on housing. Staying with relatives, which can result in overcrowding, is associated with not only physical ailments but also significant psychologic distress. Multiple moves are also associated with negative health outcomes in children. Health care providers often focus on screening for homelessness, but do not probe further to identify housing instability. It is important to assess for housing instability, as it has clearly been linked with poor health outcomes. Based on recent estimates, approximately 50% of the homeless youth in America identify as a member of the lesbian, gay, bisexual, transgender (LGBT) community.

Case 9 answers

Q 9.1: b. Social gradient

This is an example of social gradient in health. It is well established that those with low socioeconomic status suffer from poorer health than those higher on the social ladder. The social gradient affects all members of society, such that though they have many more resources, middle class individuals still suffer from poorer health than upper class individuals. An understanding of social structures and norms may help inform solutions to closing this societal gap.

Suggested further readings

1. Healthypeople.gov. Quality of housing. <https://www.healthypeople.gov/2020/topics-objectives/topic/social-determinants-health/interventions-resources/quality-of-housing>; Accessed 21.03.18.
2. Cockerham WC, Hamby BW, Oates GR. The social determinants of chronic disease. *Am J Prev Med*. 2017;52: S5-S12.
3. Wilkinson R, Marmot M. Social gradient. In: Wilkinson R, Marmot M, eds. *Social Determinants of Health: The Solid Facts*. 2nd ed. Denmark: World Health Organization; 2003.

Case 10 answers

Q 10.1: b. Access to health care

Though all these factors likely play a role in Mr. Harris's COPD, access to health care is the least likely to have contributed to his recent admission. Occupational exposures, poverty, and environmental exposures have all shown a high association with the development and/or severity of COPD. Access to health care plays a role; however, studies have shown that when access to health care is equal, populations with lower socioeconomic status still experience worse health outcomes.

Q 10.2: a. Health inequality

This is an example of health inequality, or "differences in health status or in the distribution of health determinants between different population groups." In contrast, health care disparity refers to differences in access to care. Interventions aimed toward preventing the development or progression of COPD in populations with low socioeconomic status seek to achieve health equity.

Q 10.3: a. Community-based smoking cessation classes

Data regarding the efficacy of community-based smoking cessation classes is mixed. If successful, smoking cessation would be the most effective strategy in preventing symptoms and poor health outcomes from COPD for Mr. Harris. However, early education and primary prevention would be ideal to decrease the rate of smoking in young people within the community. Though removing the exposure to mold and improving the likelihood of medication adherence would both be beneficial, neither would be as efficacious as smoking cessation. A multifactorial approach would be the most optimal plan; however, efforts targeted toward smoking cessation in patients with COPD are likely to result in the most significant decrease in morbidity and mortality.

Suggested further reading

1. Centers for Disease Control and Prevention. NCHHSTP social determinants of health. <https://www.cdc.gov/nchhstp/socialdeterminants/definitions.html>; 2014 Accessed 21.03.18.

Case 11 answers

Q 11.1: a. Elder abuse

Social isolation is associated with substantial health risks and has been associated with increased morbidity and mortality. These health risks are particularly notable in older adults. Social isolation and depression are clearly linked. Both may contribute to the increased severity of the other. However, social isolation, independent of whether it prompts feelings of loneliness, has been associated with worse physical health. Therefore, it is imperative that we screen for social isolation in high-risk patients such as Mr. Smith. Social isolation and depression may be making it difficult for Mr. Smith to implement his care plan. In addition, access to healthy food is also likely to be contributing. Though not formally screened in this example, Mr. Smith does not demonstrate red flags for elder abuse. Nevertheless, elder abuse affects as many as 10% of older adults in the United States. Though the US Preventive Services Task Force has determined that there is insufficient evidence to make a recommendation regarding screening, many other professional organizations recommend routine screening.

Q 11.2: a. Financial security

In a survey performed by AARP (formerly the American Association of Retired Persons), 51% of adults over the age of 50 reported at least one unmet social need. A total of 23% reported that they had difficulty paying their bills or had to choose between food and other necessities. Also, 22% reported that they felt lonely often, and 16% reported that, in the past year, there was a time during which they did not have sufficient financial resources to obtain enough food. Additionally, 12% had transportation difficulties outside of the home, and 11% had difficulty getting around in their homes. Approximately 28% reported two or more unmet social needs. This highlights the importance of identifying social determinants of health that may be impacting older adults in particular.

Q 11.3: c. AAAs only serve Americans over the age of 60 years

Area Agencies on Aging receive funding through the Older Americans Act, although most AAAs also receive funding from other state and local sources. Because they are controlled at the local level, the exact services offered vary by county. All AAAs offer the following five core services:

- Elder rights, including elder abuse intervention and legal services
- Caregivers, including referral to local resources that offer in-home services
- Nutrition, such as nutrition counseling and referral to meal delivery services
- Health and wellness, particularly at senior centers, where exercise and health education programs may be available
- Supportive services, including case management and transportation services

Many AAAs provide additional services. AAAs are not limited to adults over the age of 60 years. They provide services to veterans of all ages and caregivers of older adults. In addition, they provide services to those with disabilities.

Case 12 answers

Q 12.1: d. All of the above

Programs of All-Inclusive Care for the Elderly (PACE) is a program within Medicare and Medicaid that is available in 31 states. Patients such as Mr. Smith, who are older than 55 years and require nursing home level of care, can receive services that are geared toward keeping them at home safely. Telemanagement systems are increasingly available for the management of multiple chronic conditions. In the case of heart failure, for example, use of electronic scales and blood pressure cuffs that automatically transmit information to providers can allow for adjustment in management strategies aimed toward preventing hospitalizations. Multiple randomized controlled trials are underway to determine the efficacy of such programs. Veterans Affairs Home Based Primary Care programs were first implemented in the 1970s but have since grown. These programs serve as the primary care providers for veterans who are chronically ill with complex comorbidities. They aim to maximize veteran independence while preventing hospitalization. Mr. Smith may benefit from any one of these services.

Suggested further readings

1. Pooler J, Liu S, Roberts A. *Older adults and unmet social needs: prevalence and health implications.* AARP Foundation. <http://endseniorhunger.aarp.org/wp-content/uploads/2017/11/SDOH-among-older-adults-2017_IssueBrief_COR-Final.pdf>; 2017 Accessed 21.03.18.
2. Area Agencies on Aging. Local leaders in aging and community living. <https://www.n4a.org/Files/LocalLeadersAAA2017.pdf>; 2017 Accessed 21.03.18.
3. National Research Council (US) Panel on a Research Agenda and New Data for an Aging World. *Preparing for an Aging World: The Case for Cross-National Research.* Vol. 6. Washington, DC: National Academies Press; 2001.
4. Medicare.gov. PACE. <https://www.medicare.gov/your-medicare-costs/get-help-paying-costs/pace>; Accessed 02.04.18.

Case 13 answers

Q 13.1: d. Of children who are food insecure, 20% come from families that do not qualify for federal nutrition assistance programs

Food insecurity is defined as lack of consistent access to adequate food. Another definition adds that limited access may be due to cost, but also due to proximity to food sources and/or other resources. The US Department of Agriculture estimates that 41 million people are affected by food insecurity in the United States—14 million of those affected are children. The rates of food insecurity in the United States have been trending down since 2009 (from 15.4% in 2014 to 13.4% in 2015). Though this is encouraging, the weekly food budget shortfall, or reported amount of money needed for food per week, by food insecure individuals, is rising. Unfortunately, up to 26% of those dealing with food insecurity also have annual incomes that disqualify them from federal nutrition assistance programs.

Food deserts are defined as follows:

- In urban areas, access to a supermarket within 1 mile of home
- In rural areas, access to a supermarket within 10 miles of home

Q 13.2: a. Development of heart disease as an adult

Childhood obesity rates in the United States from 2011 to 2014 were estimated to be around 17%. Being overweight or obese during childhood is linked to multiple short- and long-term complications. Children with obesity are more likely to be obese as adults, compared to their normal weight counterparts. In addition, they are at risk for developing all of the following complications:

- Asthma
- Sleep apnea
- Bone and joint problems
- Type 2 diabetes
- Heart disease
- Cancers such as esophageal adenocarcinoma, colon cancer, renal cancer, and endometrial cancer (though obesity has been linked to multiple cancers, lung cancer is not noted to be more prevalent in obese individuals)
- Childhood social isolation, bullying, and depression

Q 13.3: a. In the last 12 months, how often have you been worried that food would run out before you got money to buy more?

Multiple screening tools have been used by providers to identify patients at risk for food insecurity. In particular, a two-question screen has been shown to be highly predictive of food insecurity. A large study in 2010 revealed that an affirmative answer to either question was 97% sensitive and 83% specific for accurately identifying food insecurity.

In the past 12 months, was the following statement often true, sometimes true, or never true for your household?

1. We were worried that food would run out before we got money to buy more.

2. The food we bought just didn't last, and we didn't have money to get more.

The question "Do you have difficulty making ends meet?" is an initial screening question that is often used to try to identify poverty in general but has not been validated for use in identifying food insecurity.

Q 13.4: c. A focus on strengthening assets

Though there is little doubt as to the value of identifying social determinants of health in our patient populations, screening for social determinants of health may result in inadvertent negative consequences. Employing screening tools without having the resources to address identified challenges or barriers may lead to disappointment or distrust of providers by patients. The manner in which screening occurs can also damage the therapeutic relationship. Not taking the individual patient and family situation into account, as often occurs with automatic referral processes, may be detrimental. Considering individual context and using shared decision making can help health care providers address needs or barriers in a more patient-centered manner. Screening practices that are geared toward specific demographic factors may reinforce stereotypes and further alienate patients. In contrast, such screening practices may also miss at-risk individuals whose outward characteristics may not accurately reflect their needs. When assessing patients, it is important to not only identify their gaps or needs, but also to identify their strengths. Fortifying their strengths can prove as useful as addressing their deficits.

Suggested further readings

1. Feeding American. Map the meal gap 2018. <https://www.feedingamerica.org/sites/default/files/research/map-the-meal-gap/2016/2016-map-the-meal-gap-all-modules.pdf>; 2018 Accessed 21.04.18.
2. The State of Obesity. Food insecure children. <https://stateofobesity.org/food-insecurity/>; Accessed 21.04.18.
3. Centers for Disease Control and Prevention. Childhood obesity facts. <https://www.cdc.gov/healthyschools/obesity/facts.htm>; 2018 Accessed 02.04.18.
4. Andermann A. Taking action on the social determinants of health in clinical practice: a framework for health professionals. *CMAJ*. 2016;188:E474-E483.
5. Garg A, Boynton-Jarrett R, Dworkin PH. Avoiding the unintended consequences of screening for social determinants of health. *JAMA*. 2016;316(8):813-814.

5

Population and Public Health

Rachel Apple, MD, MPH, Sophia Kostelanetz, MD, MPH

Cases and questions

Case 1

Dr. Samuel Jones is a family medicine physician in the Midwest. He recently joined a private practice group associated with an accountable care organization. He anticipates being responsible for the care of approximately 1800 patients, ranging in age from birth to over 90 years old, predominantly in the outpatient primary care setting. His practice accepts most types of health insurance and specializes in providing comprehensive care for patients with diabetes and hyperlipidemia.

Q 1.1: The health outcomes of a group of individuals, including the distribution of health outcomes within the group, refer to what type of health?
a. Public health
b. Population health
c. Individualized health
d. Socialized health
e. Community health

Q 1.2: As Dr. Jones considers his new role, which of the following groups represents potential populations that could be defined within his patient panel?
a. Patients with diabetes mellitus
b. Patients with a particular type of health insurance
c. Patients who identify at lesbian, gay, bisexual, transgender (LGBT)
d. Patients who live in a particular zip code near the clinic
e. None of the above
f. All of the above

Q 1.3: Based upon the information provided, which of the four major pillars of population health is already a focus within Dr. Jones's practice?
a. Chronic care management
b. Quality and safety
c. Public health
d. Health policy
e. Both a and c

Case 2

One of Dr. Jones's partners in the practice wants to start a new initiative focused on increased utilization of a new medication to treat obesity. The partner tells Dr. Jones that this medication will help many of their patients who have obesity, diabetes, and hyperlipidemia.

Q 2.1: Dr. Jones is interested in helping his patients, but he recalls that the overall health of a population results from a complex interplay of determinants of health. Which determinant of population health typically has the greatest impact on a given population?
a. Genetics
b. Health care
c. Social circumstances
d. Behavior
e. Environmental exposures

Q 2.2: What percent of determinants of population health is attributed to medical care?
a. 10%
b. 20%
c. 30%
d. 40%
e. 50%

Case 3

Dr. Kimberly Smith is a physician who works for her state department of health at a community-based health clinic. She is interested in improving her community's rates of childhood vaccination and decreasing the rates of sexually transmitted infections, including human immunodeficiency virus (HIV). Her state health department recently started an initiative focused on reducing lead and carbon monoxide exposure within the community. Dr. Smith is interested in learning about the prevalence of HIV in her state. She references the Behavioral Risk Factor Surveillance System (BRFSS) data to determine the state-based prevalence of HIV in her state.

Q 3.1: Use of BRFSS data is an example of which core function of public health?
a. Policy development
b. Assurance
c. Assessment
d. Evaluation
e. Education

Q 3.2: Dr. Smith decides that she wants to design a study utilizing the BRFSS data to compare HIV prevalence among various demographic and geographic populations throughout her state. She plans to use the outcomes from this study to inform her next outreach initiative focused on educating the local community about HIV. This is an example of which public health essential services?
a. Evaluation, diagnosis, investigation, and law enforcement
b. Policy development, mobilization of community partnerships, and education
c. Research, system management, and assurance of competent workforce
d. Provision of care, health monitoring, and evaluation
e. Evaluation, research, and education

Q 3.3: Which of the following is NOT a true statement regarding population health and public health?
a. Public health is one of the four pillars of population health
b. Population health is built on public health fundamentals, especially disease prevention and health promotion
c. Public health is primarily community based
d. Population health is more directly connected to government health departments than public health
e. Population health reaches more broadly into the health care delivery arena than public health

Q 3.4: Dr. Smith is seeing one of her patients who was recently admitted to the hospital for an acute coronary syndrome. He was discharged from the hospital 5 days ago and presents today for follow-up. Dr. Smith does not have access to any of this patient's records from the recent admission. The patient does not have a list of his discharge medications and is unsure of his current medication list. This scenario is an example of which type of limitation of the current US health system?
a. Focus on sick care over prevention and wellness
b. Siloed and fragmented efforts for health and health care

c. Inadequate assimilation and use of data
d. Suboptimal patient engagement
e. Inequality and inequity in health and health outcomes
f. Both b and c
g. All of the above

Q 3.5: Which of the five core disciplines of public health is the focus of the health department's new initiative?
a. Epidemiology
b. Biostatistics
c. Environmental health sciences
d. Social and behavioral sciences
e. Health policy and management

Case 4

Bridgette is a second-year medical student who is doing an away rotation at the Centers for Disease Control and Prevention. During her rotation, she is asked to develop an initiative focused on one of the five key areas identified by Healthy People 2020. She decides to focus her proposal on developing an after-school program for elementary-aged children, which aims to reduce gang-related violence.

Q 4.1: Which of the five key areas of Healthy People 2020 is the main focus of Bridgette's project?
a. Economic stability
b. Education
c. Social and community context
d. Health and health care
e. Neighborhood and built environment

Case 5

Dr. Williams is a family physician at a large academic center in Chicago. In his primary care practice, he sees children and adults. In reviewing his patient panel, he notices a trend toward higher body mass indices (BMIs) and hemoglobin A1c levels for his diabetic patients who live in a particular neighboring zip code. After noticing this trend, he investigates further and finds that this zip code also has the highest rate of infant mortality and gun-related deaths in the city.

Q 5.1: What term best describes the variation in health outcomes that Dr. Williams notices among his patient panel?
a. Health inaccuracies
b. Health disparities
c. Health discrepancies
d. Health inequities
e. Both b and d

Q 5.2: If incorporated into his practice, which of the following initiatives would exemplify a focus on meeting the goals set forth in the Triple Aim?
a. The practice would survey its patients regarding their experience with clinic staff and physicians
b. The practice would engage in quality improvement projects aimed at reducing wasted resources in the clinic and increasing efficiency
c. The practice would use a dashboard to monitor the hemoglobin A1c levels of all the patients with diabetes

d. Both a and c

e. All of the above

Q 5.3: What term applies to a primary care model that provides comprehensive, team-based, patient-centered, coordinated, accessible care focused on quality and patient safety?

a. Accountable care organization

b. Hospital managed organization

c. Academic medical center

d. Patient-centered medical home

e. Walk-in clinic

Case 6

Ms. Reed is a 45-year-old single lesbian woman who is overweight and has a history of poorly controlled diabetes. She lives alone, spends much of her time watching television, and does not have a license to drive a car. She rarely sees her doctor and has never had a cervical cancer screening test because she is only sexually active with women. She is admitted for a severe upper respiratory infection and spends 3 days in the hospital receiving intravenous antibiotics. After stabilization, she is set up with home nursing services and discharged home with a plan for follow-up with a case manager.

Q 6.1: With a new case manager assigned to her care postdischarge, the affordable care organization hopes to overcome which of the following limitations in the US health system?

a. Focus on sick care

b. Siloed and fragmented efforts of health and health care

c. Inadequate simulation and use of data

d. Suboptimal patient engagement

e. All of the above

f. None of the above

Q 6.2: Ms. Reed's obesity and poorly controlled diabetes put her at risk for further complications leading to increased morbidity and mortality. You overhear someone state that if only Ms. Reed ate healthier and exercised, instead of watching television all day and eating junk, she would not have any of these problems. You agree that patient engagement is important. What other considerations would you suggest could be playing a role?

a. Nothing, as Ms. Reed is simply lazy and her health outcomes are her own fault

b. You would recommend evaluating her access to healthy food, transportation, and home and neighborhood environments

c. Because prior studies have shown the combined cost of health inequalities and premature deaths in the United States between 2003 and 2006 to be $1.24 trillion, you would recommend evaluating the social determinants of health that could be contributing to her poor health

d. Because adults who identify as lesbian, gay, bisexual (LGB) are twice as likely as heterosexual adults to suffer from anxiety or depression, you would recommend evaluating Ms. Reed for depression as a barrier to increased patient engagement

e. Choices b, c, and d

f. Both b and d

g. None of the above

Q 6.3: As discussed in this chapter, which of the following practices would reflect a function of managing population health that would be an improvement over the prior individual care model?

a. Ms. Reed's primary care physician will titrate Ms. Reed's insulin to optimize her diabetes management

b. Ms. Reed's primary care physician will refer her to ophthalmology to screen for and prevent diabetes-associated eye conditions

c. Ms. Reed's primary care physician will refer her to social work after finding that Ms. Reed has no access to transportation for her ophthalmology appointment

d. Ms. Reed's primary care physician will ensure she has appropriate vaccinations to decrease the risk of influenza

Q 6.4: Known and well-documented health disparities in America include which of the following?

a. Life expectancy disparity among races

b. Infant mortality disparity among races

c. Diabetes prevalence by gender, race, education, and socioeconomic class

d. Food deserts preventing access to healthy food for the poor

e. All of the above

f. None of the above

Q 6.5: Which of the following is NOT related to health disparities, as defined by Healthy People 2020?

a. Social

b. Genetic

c. Economic

d. Environmental

e. None of the above

Q 6.6: Which of the following is NOT true about a community health needs assessment (CHNA)?

a. It is a process that uses quantitative and qualitative methods to systematically collect and analyze data to understand health within a specific community

b. Health care organizations collaborate with community residents and organizations to complete a CHNA

c. The data are used to inform community decision making, the prioritization of health problems, and the development, implementation, and evaluation of community health improvement plans

d. The Affordable Care Act required for-profit hospitals to perform a CHNA every 3 years

Q 6.7: Which of the following is NOT true about accountable care organizations (ACOs)?

a. An ACO is a model of primary care that provides comprehensive, team-based, patient-centered, coordinated, accessible care that is focused on quality and patient safety

b. An ACO is an integrated system of health care professionals/organizations in a formal agreement with a payer to care for a defined patient population

c. ACOs are accountable for cost, quality, and outcomes of its population of patients

d. ACOs may be accountable for losses and repayment to Medicare if patient care expenditures exceed certain benchmarks

Q 6.8: For which of the following programs are hospitals eligible for value-based incentive payments measured by clinical processes of care, patient experience, and outcomes?
a. Bundled payments
b. Value-based purchasing
c. The Hospital Readmission Reduction Program
d. The Hospital Acquired Condition Reduction Program
e. All of the above

Case 7

You are working at a consulting firm hired by your local hospital to increase value during inpatient hospitalizations. The hospital leadership would like to improve quality but is most concerned about addressing quality concerns that could lead to penalties.

Q 7.1: Which of the following interventions could prevent Medicare penalties to the local hospital?
a. An intervention to decrease unnecessary daily labs and imaging in hospitalized patients, starting with those on units with total knee arthroplasties that are part of the bundled payment program
b. An intervention to improve patient satisfaction in an effort to improve ratings on *Hospital Compare* and thus improve value-based payments
c. An intervention to ensure better outpatient follow-up coordination and medication reconciliation for patients with heart failure exacerbations and to decrease readmissions within 30 days
d. Both a and b
e. Both b and c
f. None of the above

Case 8

You are invited to participate in a hackathon for health care. A local primary care clinic in Boston has asked for solutions for improving diabetes management in its poorest populations.

Q 8.1: One of your colleagues suggests that using an electronic health record (EHR) in all of the clinics will invariably improve all aspects of diabetes management. What would be the best response?
a. "I agree! If we had more timely and efficient access to patient data, our patients would have perfect diabetes management. If providers knew the blood glucose numbers for all of their patients, they would be able to overcome all the hurdles with diabetes management."
b. "I somewhat agree! An EHR would improve some aspects of management. However, I am worried that we would need to include other interventions, as EHRs often do not include retrievable data on determinants of health."
c. "I disagree! An EHR is a complete waste of money. They do not improve the ability for population or patient management."
d. "I disagree! Only primary care physicians can access the EHR, which would make it hard for the nurses, technicians, and dieticians to participate in care."

Q 8.2: One of the challenges to improved diabetes management is ensuring that patients have regular follow-up and access to subspecialists when needed (ophthalmology, podiatry, etc). The hackathon challenges you to improve access to care for these patients. Which of the following would NOT accomplish that goal?
a. Employing telemedicine to improve access to subspecialists for patients in rural areas via their primary care sites
b. Employing a community health worker to visit patients in their homes or at work, whichever is acceptable to the patient
c. Implementing a patient portal to improve communication between providers and patients
d. Implementing a patient portal to allow patients to seek urgent and emergent care when needed (i.e., for severe hypoglycemia or hyperglycemia)
e. All of the above

Q 8.3: One of the hackathon groups proposes using a Camden Coalition model to improve diabetes care for poor populations. Which of the following statements is NOT true about the Camden Coalition of Healthcare Providers?
a. The Camden Coalition's key initiative is to change national policy to support decreased smoking, sodium intake, and trans-fat consumption
b. The Camden Coalition is a coalition of hospitals, primary care providers, and community representatives who collaborate to deliver better health care to vulnerable citizens
c. The Camden Coalition uses a technique called "hot spotting" to geographically identify high-need areas for high-utilizer patients to improve access to care
d. A key aspect of the intervention is to use a multidisciplinary team to visit the patient, both in and out of the hospital

Answers

Case 1 answers

Q 1.1: b. Population health
Population health is defined as the health outcomes of a group of individuals, including the distribution of health outcomes within the group. Population health extends beyond the individual patient focus and encompasses health outcomes of groups, communities, or populations of individuals. Public health is defined as "[w]hat we as a society do collectively to assure the conditions in which people can be healthy." Public health is one of the four major pillars of population health and is a discipline focusing on the health of specific groups. Public health has not traditionally focused on individual medical care or private sector health care delivery. Individualized health relates to the attempt to personalize or individualize health care delivery for a given person or group of people. Community health is a term often used to refer to the health system in a given community and/or efforts aimed at health care delivery in a specific, localized population.

Q 1.2: f. All of the above
All of these are examples of populations that could be defined within Dr. Jones's practice. Populations may be defined in multiple ways. Examples of populations include individuals in a specific geographic area or community, underserved individuals who share a common

characteristic (i.e., ethnic or sexual minorities), patients with a specific medical condition, or individuals in a certain health insurance plan.

Q 1.3: a. Chronic care management

Dr. Jones's practice is already focusing on comprehensive management of diabetes mellitus and hyperlipidemia, two chronic medical conditions. His practice should also work to incorporate the other three pillars of population health: public health, quality and safety, and health policy. The four major pillars of population health are chronic care management, quality and safety, public health, and health policy. As population health is strongly focused on analysis of outcomes to drive process change and new policies, we can use various frameworks to help conceptualize the interplay between the four pillars and outcomes. In the framework shown in Fig. 5.1, we see that the health outcomes of a population (i.e., population health) are the result of a complex interplay of determinants of health, policies, and programs. Chronic medical conditions, quality and safety, public health, and health policy factor into this complex relationship on multiple levels.

Case 2 answers

Q 2.1: d. Behavior

Only about 10% of the determinants of population health are attributed to medical care. The vast majority of population health determinants are related to behavior or lifestyle choices, social circumstances, and environmental exposures. While a medication may help some of the practice's patients with obesity, diabetes, and hyperlipidemia, examining the behaviors, social circumstances, and environmental factors that influence the population of patients with these chronic illnesses would be a more appropriate first step (Fig. 5.2).

Q 2.2: a. 10%

Despite medical care being the predominant focus in the health arena in the United States, only 10% of

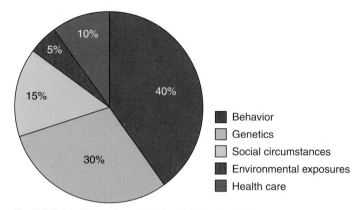

Fig. 5.2 Determinants of population health. (Data from McGinnis JM, Williams-Russo P, Knickman JR. The case for more active policy attention to health promotion. *Health Aff* [Millwood]. 2002;21[2]:78-93.).

determinants of population health are attributable to medical care. As demonstrated in Fig. 5.2, the majority of population health determinants fall into the category of behavior or lifestyle choices (40%), genetics (30%), or social circumstances (15%). From a population health perspective, there is motivation for new strategies that take into account the impenetrable link between a person's health status and his or her home, work, school, or other environments, rather than focusing strictly on his or her interaction with the health system directly.

Case 3 answers

Q 3.1: c. Assessment

Public health has three core functions and ten essential services. The three core functions are assessment, assurance, and policy development. Use of BRFSS data is an example of the assessment function of the public health system (Fig. 5.3). In its assessment function, public health agencies monitor health status to identify and solve community health problems and diagnose

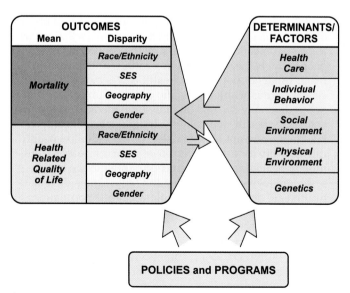

Fig. 5.1 The four major pillars of population health. (Kindig DA. University of Wisconsin Population Health. What Are Population Health Determinants or Factors?)

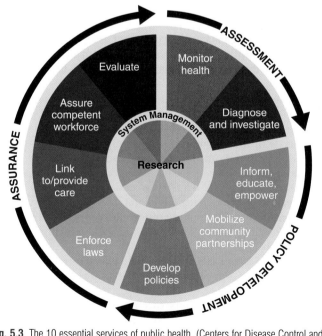

Fig. 5.3 The 10 essential services of public health. (Centers for Disease Control and Prevention. Office for State, Local, Tribal, and Territorial Support. NPHPS Overview)

and investigate health problems and hazards in the community. In its assurance function, public health enforces laws and regulations that protect health, and evaluates the effectiveness, accessibility, and quality of person- and population-based health services. Public health also connects people to health services when they are otherwise unavailable. In its policy development function, public health informs and educates individuals about health issues, develops polices and plans in support of individual and community health efforts, and mobilizes community partnerships to meet community health needs. Refer to Chapter 10, "Population Health," Section II "What is Population Health?" Part C "Public Health" for additional examples of each of the three core functions of public health.

Q 3.2: e. Evaluation, research, and education

Dr. Smith's study idea best encompasses the essential services of research, evaluation, and education. There are 10 essential services of public health: evaluation, assurance of competent workforce, link to/provision of care, law enforcement, policy development, mobilization of community partnerships, inform/educate/empower, diagnosis and investigation, health monitoring, and research (see Fig. 5.3). While her project could also involve elements of other essential services, it clearly addresses research and has application in the evaluation of HIV prevalence and education.

Q 3.3: d. Population health is more directly connected to government health departments than public health

Typically, public health actively monitors community health status, investigates health problem, develops programs and initiatives focused on health promotion and disease prevention, and is primarily community based. The public health system is more closely connected to government-based health departments.

Q 3.4: f. Both b and c

While all of the listed answers could have played a role in this scenario, the two most proximal limitations are siloed and fragmented care as well as inadequate assimilation and use of data. This patient has had to access many different points of care for his health care, and lack of coordination and communication between these points contributed to fragmentation of the health system. Additionally, this example demonstrates limited communication and information sharing between the various parties involved in caring for the patient. Medical care and public health data sources are often not well connected. All of the listed answers are examples of significant limitations in US health care, which must be overcome to achieve improved population health.

Q 3.5: c. Environmental health sciences

The health department's new initiative focusing on reduced exposures to lead and carbon monoxide is an example of the core discipline of environmental health sciences. The other listed options compose the remaining core disciplines of public health: epidemiology, biostatistics, social and behavioral sciences, and health policy and management. Often there is overlap between these disciplines in a given project or initiative.

Case 4 answers

Q 4.1: e. Neighborhood and built environment

Bridgette's proposal is most closely linked with the Healthy People 2020's focus on neighborhoods and the built environment as it aims to reduce crime and violence. Her project also relates to the social and community context, as it could also have a distal impact on reduction of incarceration and improving a sense of community among the residents. Healthy People 2020 is a US initiative focused on health promotion for all Americans. The five key areas targeted by Healthy People 2020 are economic stability, education, social and community context, health and health care, and the neighborhood and built environment.

Case 5 answers

Q 5.1: e. Both b and d

Differences in health and health outcomes between groups of people are considered health disparities. When differences are considered avoidable, unjust, or unfair, they are often referred to as health inequities. In this case, both terms are appropriately applied to Dr. William's patient health outcomes which vary on the basis of zip code. In this case, zip code is likely a proxy for socioeconomic status and/or race and ethnicity.

Q 5.2: e. All of the above

The Triple Aim includes a focus on improved patient experience, improved health of populations, and lower per capita cost. A patient survey is a way to understand the patient experience and potentially improve the clinic experience for patients. Quality improvement projects designed to reduce waste can facilitate lowering per capita costs on a micro or macro level. Utilization of a dashboard to monitor the glycemic control of a given population, such as the population of patients in this clinic with diabetes, is an example of improving the health of populations (Fig. 5.4).

Q 5.3: d. Patient-centered medical home

This is the definition of a patient-centered medical home (PCMH). The PCMH is a model of primary care that

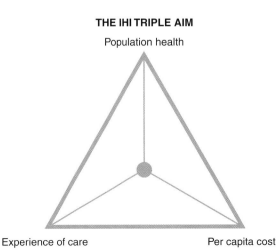

THE IHI TRIPLE AIM

Population health

Experience of care   Per capita cost

Fig. 5.4 The IHI Triple Aim framework developed by the Institute for Healthcare Improvement in Cambridge, Massachusetts (ihi.org).

provides comprehensive, team-based, patient-centered, coordinated, accessible care that is focused on quality and patient safety. It emerged in the late 1960s as a model for caring for children with special needs, but has since expanded to other populations. The Affordable Care Act has several provisions that promote the implementation of this model.

Case 6 answers

Q 6.1: e. All of the above

An accountable care organization (ACO) is an integrated system of health care professionals/organizations in a formal agreement with a payer to care for a defined population. The ACO is accountable for the quality of care, health expenditures, and outcomes for its population of patients. The new case manager, as part of the ACO, will help the patient access acute care (which he already received during his hospitalization) and follow up for chronic disease management to hopefully prevent readmissions. The case manager can also decrease fragmentation in health care and inadequate transfer of patient data by assuring the primary care physician gets discharge summaries and instructions (e.g., including laboratory tests, imaging, and new medication doses, and lists from past hospitalization). Follow-up phone calls may also help with patient engagement.

Q 6.2: e. Choices, b, c, and d

An accountable care organization (ACO) is an integrated system of health care professionals/organizations in a formal agreement with a payer to care for a defined population. The ACO is accountable for the quality of care, health expenditures, and outcomes for its population of patients. If Ms. Reed lives in a food desert with only limited nonrefrigerated packaged food at the corner store, education alone regarding eating more fresh vegetables and healthy grains and proteins is likely insufficient. There may be limited options for transportation to areas with healthier food options. She may have no sidewalks in her neighborhood. She may have concerns about violent crime that keep her from going outside. Choice c is also correct. The estimated combined cost of health inequalities and premature deaths in the mentioned studies was $1.24 trillion. Untreated or insufficiently treated mental health disease is a common barrier to improved patient engagement.

Q 6.3: c. Ms. Reed's primary care physician will refer her to social work after finding that Ms. Reed has no access to transportation for her ophthalmology appointment

In the classic individualized care model, Ms. Reed's primary care physician would titrate insulin to optimize diabetes management, refer to ophthalmology for diabetes screening and prevention, and assure appropriate vaccination. When considering the larger view of population health, Ms. Reed's primary care physician would not only consider the direct medical care Ms. Reed requires, but also the social determinants of health that may preclude her being able to access care, such as lack of transportation.

Q 6.4: e. All of the above

In Chicago the difference in life expectancy is 16 years when comparing the predominantly African American Washington Park neighborhood on the South Side to the predominantly Caucasian Loop in the city center just 5 miles away. Nationally, infant mortality remains highest for non-Hispanic black women. Diabetes prevalence is highest among males, individuals 65 years of age and older, non-Hispanic blacks and those of mixed race, Hispanics, individuals with less than a high school education, those who are poor, and those with a disability. Food deserts prevent access to healthy foods and thus are a barrier to preventive health measures.

Q 6.5: b. Genetic

Genetic predisposition is not a health disparity. A health disparity adversely affects groups of people who have systematically experienced greater obstacles to health based on their racial or ethnic group; religion; socioeconomic status; gender; age; mental health; cognitive, sensory, or physical disability; sexual orientation or gender identity; geographic location; or other characteristics historically linked to discrimination or exclusion.

Q 6.6: d. The Affordable Care Act required for-profit hospitals to perform a CHNA every 3 years

A CHNA is a "process that uses quantitative and qualitative methods to systematically collect and analyze data to understand health within a specific community. The data can inform community decision making, the prioritization of health problems, and the development, implementation, and evaluation of community health improvement plans." The Affordable Care Act required not-for-profit hospitals to perform a CHNA every 3 years to maintain their 501(c)(3) status for tax purposes.

Q 6.7: a. An ACO is a model of primary care that provides comprehensive, team-based, patient-centered, coordinated, accessible care that is focused on quality and patient safety

Q 6.8: b. Value-based purchasing

Bundled payments are set payments for services rendered during a patient's episode of care (course of treatment for a certain medical condition or illness). The Hospital Readmission Reduction Program penalizes hospitals for relatively higher Medicare readmissions. The Hospital Acquired Condition Reduction Program reduces Medicare payment to the poorest performing hospitals.

Case 7 answers

Q 7.1: c. An intervention to ensure better outpatient follow-up coordination and medication reconciliation for patients with heart failure exacerbations and to decrease readmissions within 30 days

The Hospital Admission Reduction program penalizes hospitals for relatively higher Medicare readmissions. Over the lifetime of the program, defined penalties for readmissions of specific diagnoses have evolved. For example, fiscal year 2015 penalties applied to acute myocardial infarction, heart failure, pneumonia, chronic obstructive pulmonary disease, and hip/knee arthroplasty. Choice a could help prevent wasteful imaging and laboratories but would not be associated with Medicare penalties. Choice b could improve ratings but would not be associated with Medicare penalties.

Case 8 answers

Q 8.1: b. "I somewhat agree! An EHR would improve some aspects of management. However, I am worried that we would need to include other interventions, as EHRs often do not include retrievable data on determinants of health."

While EHRs potentially improve timely and efficient access to patient data, EHRs have notable limitations for population health, including EHR systems that often do not communicate with each other and lack of access to information on contributing social determinants of health.

Q 8.2: d. Implementing a patient portal to allow patients to seek urgent and emergent care when needed (i.e., for severe hypoglycemia or hyperglycemia)

Patient portals are useful for nonurgent communication such as requests for medication refills or adjustments, but this email-like system would not be safe for urgent or emergent health needs. Choices a, b, and c would all improve access to care.

Q 8.3: a. The Camden Coalition's key initiative is to change national policy to support decreased smoking, sodium intake, and trans-fat consumption

Choice a describes the Million Hearts Initiative, which set the goal of preventing 1 million heart attacks and strokes in a five-year period (2012-2017). While this initial objective was not met, the Million Hearts Initiative has more recently updated its goals with a focus on public and population-health based efforts (more available at: https://millionhearts.hhs.gov/about-million-hearts/index.html).

Suggested further readings

1. Kindig D, Stoddart G. What is population health? *Am J Public Health*. 2003;93(3):380-383.
2. Centers for Disease Control and Prevention. National Public Health Performance Standards. The public health system and the 10 essential public health services. <http://www.cdc.gov/nphpsp/essentialservices.html>; 2017 Accessed 05.09.18.

6

Value in Health Care

Neera Agrwal, MD, PhD, Nandita Khera MD, MPH, William C. Mundell, MD, Zayd A. Razouki, MB, ChB, MS, John C. Matulis, III, DO, MPH

Cases and questions

Case 1

Practice data show high rates of antibiotic ordering for bronchitis among many providers in Dr. M's primary care clinic. While reviewing the literature on unnecessary antibiotic usage, Dr. M was surprised to learn that as many as 50% of all antibiotic prescriptions given for upper respiratory tract infections may be unnecessary.

Q1.1: Which of the following is a known contributor to unnecessary antibiotic prescribing?
a. Timely care
b. Provider perception of patient expectations for antibiotics
c. Overdiagnosis
d. Lead-time bias

Q 1.2: In discussing this issue with his colleagues, Dr. M hears other physician interviewees attribute their antibiotic ordering to having only 15 minutes to see a patient. These physicians did not feel they had adequate time to address patient concerns. Which of the following may be an effective practice level (microsystem) innovation to engage patients in optimizing the time they spend with their physician?
a. Asking patients to not ask their doctor too many questions
b. Integrating shared decision-making tools into the visit workflow
c. Offering antibiotics to patients who have previously received antibiotics for respiratory infections without seeing them in clinic
d. Having every patient complete a standardized symptom questionnaire prior to his or her appointment

Q 1.3: Which of the following health policy actions may be reducing the provision of low-value care?
a. Limiting the sale of high deductible plans on the health care exchange
b. Increasing the demonstrated community benefit of hospitals to maintain not-for-profit status
c. Facilitation of transitions to advanced payment models
d. The sale of health insurance across state lines

Case 2

Mrs. D is a 44-year-old administrative professional with a prior medical history notable for obesity and major depressive disorder. She is presenting to clinic with intermittent low back pain which she stated began after lifting boxes 1 week ago. Her pain is localized to the low back, is not radiating, and is not associated with any other symptoms. Her exam is notable for tender musculature in the lumbosacral region; neurologic exam is normal. Her physician orders a magnetic resonance image (MRI) of the lumbar spine "just to make sure there is nothing to be concerned about" that may be causing her pain.

Q 2.1: What is the most important potential harm to consider in ordering an MRI for this patient?
a. Radiation exposure
b. Identification of anatomic findings not related to patient's symptoms
c. Risk of nephrogenic systemic fibrosis
d. Additional clerical burden for clinical staff

Q 2.2: Considering the value equation, which of the following treatment plans is likely to provide greatest value to this patient?
a. Immediate initiation of potent opioid pain medications
b. Immediate referral to a spine specialist

c. Implementation of an approach considering activity modifications, gentle stretching, yoga, and core body strengthening

d. Place patient on short-term disability

Q 2.3: What should every physician consider prior to ordering an imaging test that may provide low-value care?

a. The pretest probability of the disease in question is for that individual patient

b. Whether imaging may be required for future referrals or for disability evaluation

c. How the decision to order a test may affect patient experience scores

d. How ordering that test may affect publicly reported quality metrics or overall cost of care

Q 2.4: What initial steps should a practice leader take to help individual physicians reduce overuse of imaging?

a. Distribute copies of guidelines on imaging for low back pain

b. Increase administrative steps, so it is more difficult to order MRIs for patients

c. Work with others to identify systemic barriers to providing high-value care

d. Ask colleagues in neurosurgery to order fewer MRIs as it may be modeling poor practice patterns for the rest of the clinic

Case 3

Mrs. W, who is 78 years old and has diagnoses of diabetes mellitus, hypertension, and Parkinson's disease, has been feeling poorly for the last week, with symptoms of cough, fever, and shortness of breath. She calls her primary care physician's office who directs her to the emergency department (ED) for further care. In the ED, Mrs. W is diagnosed with severe community-acquired pneumonia within 4 hours of arrival and is admitted to the hospital. While in the hospital, she is managed by the hospitalist with guideline-concordant antibiotics. After 3 days, she is believed to be stable enough to be discharged home on oral antibiotics. Unfortunately, 1 day after discharge, Mrs. W sustains a fall at home and calls emergency medical services to bring her back to the hospital. Upon arrival, she reports not taking her antibiotics due to her inability to get out of bed. She also tells the ED nurses that she lives alone and has run out of her other medications because she has been unable to pick up refills due to her illness.

Q 3.1: Which of the following statements is NOT correct regarding Mrs. W's course of care in the hospital?

a. Mrs. W's care has been mediated by multiple macrosystems, which include her primary care physician, the ED, and the hospitalist

b. Mrs. W's care has been mediated by multiple microsystems, which include her primary care physician, the ED, and the hospitalist

c. Mrs. W's return to the ED was most likely a result of the lack of engagement of a multidisciplinary team for discharge

d. Mrs. W had a 20% risk of readmission to the hospital within 30 days after this hospitalization for pneumonia

Q 3.2: Which of the following is a cause of ineffective transitions of care?

a. An integrated health system between the community and the health care team

b. Caregiver absence during discharge planning

c. Standardized and multidisciplinary planning and risk assessment

d. Follow-up and support at home after a patient is discharged

Q 3.3: Which of the following high-value care goals, as defined by the National Academy of Medicine (formerly the Institute of Medicine), was most likely NOT met in this patient's care?

a. Effective

b. Timely

c. Patient centered

d. Equitable

Q 3.4: Which of the following statements is correct regarding value in health care?

a. Higher health care costs are highly correlated with higher value for patients and health systems

b. All stakeholders can define value using identical or similar metrics

c. Health care payment has traditionally been based on the value of the services received by the patient

d. The lowest cost of care almost always provides the highest value for all stakeholders, including patients

e. Health care payment has traditionally been based on the number of services provided to patients

Case 4

A 43-year-old female with morbid obesity, hypertension, diabetes mellitus, and a known history of cirrhosis due to previous alcohol use is admitted with unremitting abdominal pain for 2 weeks. She was previously hospitalized at another hospital 2 days prior and was discharged home with outpatient follow-up. However, she comes to another institution because of ongoing abdominal pain that has not changed in the last 2 days. On examination, she is anxious but afebrile, and her abdominal exam reveals normal bowel sounds, diffuse pain, and no evidence of alarming peritoneal symptoms. Her laboratory studies reveal a normal white cell count (6.8×10^9/L), chronic stable anemia (9.2 g/dL), and thrombocytopenia (128×10^9/L). The liver function tests reveal a mildly elevated alkaline phosphatase (150 U/L) and normal alanine aminotransferase/aspartate transaminase (ALT/AST) and serum lipase. Her abdominal X-ray reveals normal gas pattern, with no evidence of obstruction or free air. The physician at the second hospital is able to obtain outside results from the first hospital and learns that she had a normal computed tomography (CT) scan 3 days ago, and no evidence of ascites on the ultrasound exam done there. The patient is admitted to the hospitalist service for pain control.

Q 4.1: Which of the following interventions would provide the best high-value care intervention for this patient at this time?

a. Repeating the abdominal CT scan

b. Discharging the patient with a 7-day course of opioid medications

c. Ordering daily laboratory studies to monitor the anemia and thrombocytopenia
d. Ensuring that the patient's hepatologist and primary care physician are updated with details of the patient's hospitalization

Case 5

A 50-year-old female, with a history of premature menopause, is admitted to the hospital after she fell off her horse and sustained a traumatic left hip fracture. She tells the physician that her only other medical problem is chronic anemia. She is physically very active; she can easily exert more than 4 metabolic equivalents (METS), and does so routinely in her twice-weekly cycling class. She denies any fevers, weight loss, shortness of breath, chest pain, abdominal pain, or dysuria. She takes no medications other than acetaminophen as needed, and a daily calcium supplement. She has a primary care physician, and had her laboratory studies and a screening colonoscopy done 3 months ago. Her screening mammogram was normal 6 months ago. The orthopedic surgery service asks the internist on call to provide a preoperative medical evaluation.

Q 5.1: Which of the following preoperative testing strategies would provide the highest value for the patient?
a. Electrocardiogram and chest X-ray
b. Chest X-ray and urinalysis
c. Liver function tests and complete blood count
d. Complete blood count
e. Obtain the previous laboratory studies from the primary care provider

Case 6

Mr. E is a 69-year-old male being seen by Dr. J in a primary care clinic. He has a history of hypertension, poorly controlled insulin-dependent diabetes mellitus, congestive heart failure, atrial fibrillation, and severe chronic obstructive pulmonary disease (COPD) with a forced expiratory volume per 1 second (FEV1) of 45% and diffused capacity of the lungs for carbon monoxide (DLCO) of 43%. He has smoked a pack a day since 13 years of age and quit last year after he was hospitalized 1 month for pneumonia and a COPD exacerbation. Dr. J discusses the risks and benefits of low-dose CT scan to be used for screening of lung cancer with Mr. E.

Q 6.1: Which of the following is false when considering the value of this preventive strategy?
a. Due to competing medical conditions and low potential for surviving lung cancer surgery in case of a malignancy being found, value of low-dose CT screening in this patient may be low
b. The value of this strategy is likely to be low since the patient stopped smoking last year
c. A multidisciplinary approach to screening, including radiology, pulmonary medicine, pathology, thoracic surgery, medical and radiation oncology, and other related health care disciplines is essential to enhance the value of this strategy
d. Downstream costs of screening need to be considered when evaluating the value of this strategy

Case 7

Choosing Wisely is a national campaign that aims to provide high-value care that is nonduplicative, evidence based, and reduces harm and overuse.

Q 7.1: Which of the following is NOT a potential barrier to adopting these guidelines in routine practice?
a. Patient knowledge, attitudes, and beliefs
b. Payment reforms to help implement clinical practice improvement initiatives
c. Providers' beliefs about patient concerns
d. Current medical malpractice system and concerns regarding medicolegal risks

Case 8

Mr. F is a 38-year-old with progressive multiple sclerosis who has been on treatment for 5 years. He is unable to go back to work because of the disability. His wife is his primary caregiver and takes care of their two young children. To provide high-value care for this patient when embarking on a new treatment regimen, his physician would need to discuss not only the medical side effects of the treatment but also the financial aspects of care.

Q 8.1: Which of the following may result in the physician's failure to address the patient's financial concerns?
a. Screening for financial harm by asking any concerns about how their medical care will be paid for
b. Directing them to readily available high-quality resources about medication costs and their insurance plans
c. Assuming copayment assistance programs and coupons resolve financial concerns
d. Discussing lower cost but equally efficacious alternatives, if any

Q 8.2: All of the following patient scenarios should be considered as triggers for early palliative care referrals, EXCEPT:
a. A 53-year-old female with newly diagnosed metastatic lung cancer
b. A 60-year-old male with severe congestive heart failure with significant symptom burden
c. A 49-year-old female with traumatic brain injury with complex family and psychosocial needs
d. A 30-year-old male with acute low back pain who has not seen his primary care physician for the last year

Q 8.3: Big Data has the potential to improve delivery of value-based care through which of the following means?
a. Helping identify and develop interventions to bend the cost curve for the potentially high-cost patients
b. Overrelying on electronic systems
c. Raising privacy and security issues when linking disparate data sources
d. Delivering information directly to payers so that they can be restrictive to whom they offer insurance

Case 9

A 65-year-old previously healthy woman presents with an episode of syncope after spending time training for a marathon.

She lost consciousness after standing up quickly and woke up immediately according to a standby witness. In the emergency department (ED), her blood pressure sitting was 90/40 and heart rate 105. She denies chest pain, palpitation, or shortness of breath. In the ED, an electrocardiogram (ECG) showed an elevated J point in anterior leads V1 to V3. An old ECG from 2 years ago showed similar findings. She received intravenous (IV) fluids. A cardiac stress test was negative, and the patient was discharged home.

Q 9.1: Ordering a cardiac stress test to evaluate syncope in this case is more consistent with which of the following examples?
a. Medical fraud, where the hospital filed dishonest health care claims to turn a profit
b. A missed opportunity to provide appropriate medical care when initial ECG showed ST elevation
c. Inefficiency in delivering medical care where the stress test should have been ordered prior to starting IV fluids
d. Unnecessary care where eliminating a service would not have changed the quality of care

Case 10

The rate of ordering brain computed tomography (CT) in your emergency department is 75% in patients with mild traumatic brain injury while only 15% have an acute finding on images when ordered. As part of a task force, you decide to implement a guideline-based clinical decision support intervention in your current electronic health record to reduce waste and increase value.

Q 10.1: What does available literature indicate about such interventions?
a. They are not likely to reduce rates of unnecessary imaging (i.e., waste)
b. They cause little harm and usually have no unintended consequences in the future
c. They are less successful if implemented in a large integrated health care system
d. They are more successful if the implementation strategy includes audit and feedback

Case 11

As a medical director, you receive a grant to implement an outpatient disease management project to improve health care value for the type 2 diabetes mellitus population in your clinic. Your objectives are to improve the quality of their glycemic control and reduce their health care utilization cost.

Q 11.1: When designing your intervention you should consider which of the following issues?
a. Implementing a single intervention strategy as opposed to a multifaceted strategy to reduce the cost of the intervention
b. Limiting your intervention to target poorly controlled type 2 diabetes mellitus patients to maximize the value of your intervention
c. Planning the intervention for a short period of time before the funding of your grant expires
d. Expanding your intervention to target all type 2 diabetes mellitus patients in the clinic, regardless of the severity

of their glucose control to maximize the value of your intervention

Case 12

You are part of a debate on the merits of expanding services for stroke patients. One argument is that spending more money may improve the quality of care, while others argue there is no clear association between spending more money and better health outcomes.

Q 12.1: Which of the following statements is true?
a. The evidence supports a positive, linear association between the amount of dollars spent and the quality of care
b. The evidence supports a negative linear association between the amount of dollars spent and the quality of care
c. Evidence supports that there is only a positive statistical and not a clinical association between the amount of money spent and the quality of care
d. The evidence suggests that the association between health care cost and quality is poorly understood

Case 13

A 65-year-old, low-income African American woman with a history of poorly controlled hypertension and type 2 diabetes presents to her primary care provider for a follow-up visit. She admits that she does not take her medication regularly since it is difficult to get an appointment with her primary care provider, and she has to pay significant copays for her prescriptions.

Q 13.1: Metrics assessing quality of care provided in the outpatient setting show lower scores for racial minorities and low-income populations in the following domains, EXCEPT:
a. Patient experience of care
b. Access to preventive care
c. Chronic disease management
d. Use of behavioral health services

Case 14

G.M. is a 67-year-old man with a new diagnosis of squamous cell cancer of the mouth. He has discussed various treatment options with his primary care provider, a surgeon, a medical oncologist, and a radiation oncologist. During these encounters, he asked several questions concerning his quality of life with treatment.

Q 14.1: Which of the following statements does not incorporate utility function(s) as an aid for determining value?
a. Swallowing is better preserved with cetuximab, an epidermal growth factor receptor (EGFR) inhibitor, added to chemotherapy compared with chemotherapy alone
b. Sequential treatment regimens with radiation following chemotherapy may produce less dryness of the mouth than alternating (concurrent) chemoradiation treatments
c. Patients treated with a chemotherapy regimen of docetaxel-5FU-cisplatin (TPF) showed a greater response

of metastatic lesions compared to patients treated with other chemotherapy regimens

d. Pain is better controlled when recurrence is treated with afatinib, a blocker of angiogenesis, compared to treatment with methotrexate

Case 15

Ms. G is a 75-year-old woman who is newly diagnosed with neovascular age-related macular degeneration. In discussions with her ophthalmologist, she is weighing which treatment option will be best for her.

Q 15.1: Which of the following statements or questions from the patient best demonstrates that the patient is assessing value according to value-based medicine standards?

a. "I am planning to live to age 90, so I'll go along with whatever you recommend."

b. "My cousin has diabetes and had laser treatment that worked very well. Can I expect the same for me?"

c. "What have your other patients who have my condition chosen for treatment?"

d. "Doctor, if you were in my position, which treatment would you choose?"

Case 16

Mr. F is a 40-year-old who presents to the emergency department (ED) with shortness of breath. The ED physician calculates his risk using the Wells Criteria for Pulmonary Embolism. The calculation suggests the risk of pulmonary embolism is low, but she is concerned because she missed the diagnosis of this condition in a young patient recently. She orders a CT pulmonary angiogram (CTPA) to be sure Mr. F does not have a pulmonary embolism.

Q 16.1: Of the following interventions, which is least likely to help this physician avoid unnecessary testing in the future?

a. Comparison with her peers regarding the percent of CTPAs that she orders that are positive for pulmonary embolism

b. Review of the records from her hospital of all 40-year-old men with pulmonary embolism

c. Utilize an electronic health record (EHR) decision support tool aimed to decrease the number of unnecessary diagnostic imaging orders

d. Review the meaning of a low probability score using Wells criteria

Q 16.2: Bias plays an important role in medical decision making. One's biases can lead to overtesting or undertesting. Which bias was most likely influencing Mr. F's physician to order the CTPA?

a. Availability bias

b. Optimism bias

c. Anchoring bias

d. Outcome bias

Case 17

Your institution is launching a project to reduce the cost of care for elective knee replacements. You have been identified as having expertise and training in Six Sigma methodologies. You are also known as one who keeps up on the trends to understand new approaches to these types of problems.

Q 17.1: Which of the following holds promise to broadly evaluate ways to understand and improve the value/cost equation?

a. Implementing a program to make the SOAP-V note format the standard at your institution

b. Negotiating a volume discount with the vendor of the implant preferred by your highest volume orthopedic surgeon

c. Developing a policy that incorporates a recommendation to postpone surgery on patients with a hemoglobin A1c greater than 8, since the evidence shows that there are greater hospital costs in this population

d. Utilizing principles of time-driven, activity-based costing (TDABC) that you have seen in recent articles

e. Developing a 12-week program to enroll all patients in a weight-loss and strengthening program preoperatively as you have recently read that bariatric surgery prior to joint replacement is cost effective

Case 18

Mrs. R is a 51-year-old woman with a 10-year history of heartburn. She has been treating it with bicarbonate soda two or three times per week because medications are too expensive since she lost her insurance over a year ago. She recently read in a magazine that her risk for esophageal cancer is higher with this longstanding history. When she asks for an endoscopy to evaluate this, the physician counsels her that it is not necessary. She counters that the physician is not ordering the test because she is underinsured.

Q 18.1: There is strong evidence to support her claim that her insurance status will lead to fewer tests being ordered.

a. True

b. False

Answers

Case 1 answers

Q 1.1: b. Provider perception of patient expectations for antibiotics

Unnecessary antibiotic prescribing is a well-established, significant problem. Prescribing antibiotics for bronchitis is generally considered unnecessary and would not constitute timely care. The correct answer, provider perceptions of patient expectations, has been shown to be an important factor in unnecessary antibiotic prescribing. Overdiagnosis and lead-time bias generally refer to detection of diseases that will never become clinically significant and would not be relevant concepts in this scenario.

Suggested further readings

1. Fleming-Dutra KE, Hersh AL, Shapiro DJ, et al. Prevalence of inappropriate antibiotic prescriptions among US ambulatory care visits, 2010-2011. *JAMA.* 2016;315(17):1864-1873.

2. Ebert SC. Factors contributing to excessive antimicrobial prescribing. *Pharmacotherapy.* 2007;27(10 Pt 2):S126-S130.
3. McKay R, Mah A, Law MR, McGrail K, Patrick DM. Systematic review of factors associated with antibiotic prescribing for respiratory tract infections. *Antimicrob Agents Chemother.* 2016;60(7):4106-4118.

Q 1.2: b. Integrating shared decision-making tools into the visit workflow

Asking patients to refrain from asking too many questions would be difficult to enforce, unpopular, and likely counterproductive. Integration of patient educational and shared decision-making tools into the visit flow has been shown to improve the experience and clinical outcomes of both patients and providers, and may hold promise in this scenario. While there is potential to care for patients with upper respiratory tract infections without scheduling appointments, this approach would not address current time challenges and patient experience concerns related to brief patient encounters. Provision of additional antibiotics without assessing the patient would also worsen antibiotic misuse. While many practices ask patients to complete standardized symptom questionnaires prior to their office visit, there is little evidence that questionnaires given in a nontargeted fashion improve patient engagement.

Suggested further readings

1. Elwyn G, Frosch D, Thomson R, et al. Shared decision making: a model for clinical practice. *J Gen Intern Med.* 2012;27(10):1361-1367.
2. Hoffmann TC, Montori VM, Del Mar C. The connection between evidence-based medicine and shared decision making. *JAMA.* 2014;312(13):1295-1296.

Q 1.3: c. Facilitation of transitions to advanced payment models

The impact of the sale of high deductible health plans, increasing the community benefit and the sale of insurance across state lines on the provision of low-value care, remains uncertain. Alternative payment models were designed with the intent of reducing low-value care and have shown modest benefit in doing so. For this question, this would be the most appropriate correct answer.

Suggested further readings

1. Schwartz AL, Chernew ME, Landon BE, McWilliams JM. Changes in low-value services in year 1 of the Medicare Pioneer Accountable Care Organization Program. *JAMA Intern Med.* 2015;175(11):1815-1825.
2. McWilliams JM, Hatfield LA, Chernew ME, Landon BE, Schwartz AL. Early performance of accountable care organizations in Medicare. *N Engl J Med.* 2016;374(24):2357-2366.

Case 2 answers

Q 2.1: b. Identification of anatomic findings not related to patient's symptoms

While there are many reasons not to order an MRI in this patient, the identification of anatomic findings not related to the patient's symptoms is the best choice listed. In addition to obscuring the diagnostic process, identifying unrelated anatomic findings such as degenerative disk disease is likely to cause unnecessary alarm to the patient and lead to additional phone calls, office visits, and specialty evaluations without improving outcomes. Radiation exposure is a concern in using CT imaging, but not MRI scanning. Nephrogenic systemic fibrosis is a rare complication of contrast administration, but generally is not of concern in patients without underlying kidney disease. Additionally, most lumbar spine MRIs would be performed without the addition of gadolinium contrast. While the additional clerical burden is significant, this should not be the primary reason for withholding this scan.

Suggested further reading

1. Shabana WM, Cohan RH, Ellis JH, et al. Nephrogenic systemic fibrosis: a report of 29 cases. *AJR Am J Roentgenol.* 2008;190(3):736-741.

Q 2.2: c. Implementation of an approach considering activity modifications, gentle stretching, yoga, and core body strengthening

Short-term disability and potent analgesics can be considered in some scenarios but are not routinely recommended in uncomplicated low back pain; these interventions may cause unintended harm and contribute to excessive opioid prescribing. Referral to a spine specialist is unnecessary at this juncture while conservative management would be the best option to improve the patient's symptoms.

Suggested further readings

1. Chou R. In the clinic. Low back pain. *Ann Intern Med.* 2014;160(11):ITC6-1.
2. Maher C, Underwood M, Buchbinder R. Non-specific low back pain. *Lancet.* 2017;389(10070):736-747.

Q 2.3: a. The pretest probability of the disease in question is for that individual patient

Pretest and posttest probabilities of a particular disease state when used with likelihood ratios of particular tests allow the clinician to estimate how helpful a test will be in confirming or refuting a suspected diagnosis. Whenever possible, these odds should be applied and carefully considered, along with patient preferences, in determining whether a proposed test represents low-value care.

Whether a specialist would like imaging performed prior to referral and the impact on patient experience scores or quality metrics should not be factors in determining whether to order a test.

Suggested further readings

1. Sox Jr HC. Diagnostic decision: probability theory in the use of diagnostic tests: an introduction to critical study of the literature. *Ann Intern Med.* 1986;104(1):60-66.
2. Jaeschke R, Guyatt GH, Sackett DL. Users' guides to the medical literature. III. How to use an article about a diagnostic test. B. What are the results and will they help

me in caring for my patients? The Evidence-Based Medicine Working Group. *JAMA*. 1994;271(9):703-707.

Q 2.4: c. Work with others to identify systemic barriers to providing high-value care

Employing passive physician education without understanding the drivers of the underlying performance is unlikely to be an effective long-term strategy. More effective interventions are oriented around systems level changes and ideally lessen barriers to improve performance. While physician education may be a necessary step in improving performance, it should not be the initial action taken. There are different models that can be used to guide quality improvement efforts, but all models recommend defining and understanding the drivers of an underlying problem before proposing interventions.

Therefore, a quality improvement approach where systemic challenges and barriers are identified is the initial best approach. Making it difficult to order MRIs is not known to be effective in reducing low-value care and may create patient harm when an MRI is urgently needed. Counseling subspecialty colleagues may have unintended consequences on the relationship between the practices and would also not be an appropriate initial step.

Suggested further readings

1. Van Bokhoven MA, Kok G, Van der Weijden T. Designing a quality improvement intervention: a systematic approach. *Qual Saf Health Care*. 2003;12(3):215-220.
2. Varkey P, Reller MK, Resar RK. Basics of quality improvement in health care. *Mayo Clin Proc*. 2007;82(6):735-739.

Case 3 answers

Q 3.1: a. Mrs. W's care has been mediated by multiple macrosystems, which include her primary care physician, the ED, and the hospitalist

This patient has been seen by multiple microsystems, which are defined as those providers who have direct contact with the patient, have a direct relationship with a patient, and with whom the patient's health needs are directly exchanged. The patient can be in contact with multiple microsystems at the same time. In this case, the microsystems include the ED, the hospitalist, and the patient's primary physician. In contrast, a macrosystem is a collection of many smaller systems, but these are not in direct contact with the patient. It is important to define the level of health care system, so that quality improvements are appropriately tailored. Fig. 6.1 shows the relationship between various levels of the health care system and the patient. One of the most vulnerable times for hospitalized patients with multiple chronic illnesses is when they are discharged home. Up to 20% of hospitalized patients aged 65 years and older are readmitted within 30 days, increasing both costs and adverse patient events.

Q 3.2: b. Caregiver absence during discharge planning

Transitions of care refer to the movement of patients between health care settings and health care providers.

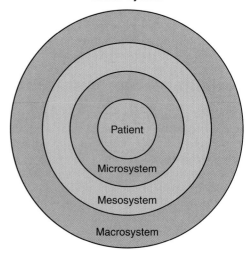

Embedded Provider Units in a Health System

Fig. 6.1 Embedded provider units in a health system. (From Nelson EC, Godfrey MM, Batalden PB, et al. Clinical microsystems, part 1. The building blocks of health systems. *Jt Comm J Qual Patient Saf*. 2008;34[7]:367-378.)

A multidisciplinary program to improve transitions of care can decrease the chance of readmissions and provide a safer environment at home for these patients. In a well-executed transition of care, caregivers must receive education, there must be clear handoffs to other providers (including the primary physician), and the patient's literacy level and understanding must be assessed and taken into account during the education process.

Q 3.3: c. Patient centered

The six domains of high-quality care as defined by the National Academy of Medicine (formerly the Institute of Medicine) are safe, timely, effective, efficient, equitable, and patient centered. This patient received guideline-concordant therapy and thus effective care, which is defined as up-to-date and guideline-based care. She also received antibiotics in a timely fashion and was treated as would any other patient, indicating timely and equitable care. However, her readmission within 1 day indicates that her care did not assess her needs and preferences. This then leads to higher costs and an overall decreased value in health care.

Q 3.4: e. Health care payment has traditionally been based on the number of services provided to patients

In the United States, the model for payment of health care services has traditionally been fee for service, thus encouraging a volume-based payment model. There is impetus to shift the payment systems to a value-based model, with institution of the Hospital Value Based Purchasing program, the Hospital Readmissions Reduction program, and implementation of the Medicare Access and CHIP Reauthorization (MACRA) program. Despite the high costs of care in the United States, there is very little evidence that the higher spending correlated with better outcomes (Fig. 6.2).

There are many stakeholders in the US health care system, including the providers, payers, the legal system, health

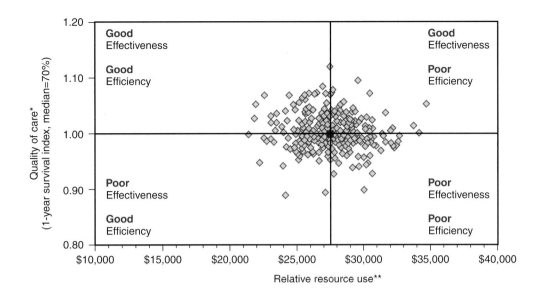

Fig. 6.2 Cost versus quality of care. (From Skochelak SE, Hawkins RE, eds. *Value in Health Care*. Philadelphia: Elsevier; 2017 [Chapter 4].)

systems, and regulatory agencies. Each of these stakeholder domains has its own definition of value that often reflects its standards rather than a patient-centric focus. Finally, while managing costs of care is important, it is also necessary to recognize that patient-centered value may sometimes be better achieved by spending more initially. Examples of this include an integrated health system that provides mental health care, multidisciplinary teams to prevent readmissions, and support after discharge home.

Suggested further readings

1. Nelson EC, Godfrey MM, Batalden PB, et al. Clinical microsystems, part 1. The building blocks of health systems. *Jt Comm J Qual Patient Saf*. 2008;34(7):367-378.
2. Merten H, Van Galen LS, Wagner C. Safe handover. *BMJ*. 2017;359:j4328.
3. Labson MC. Adapting The Joint Commision's seven foundations of safe and effective transitions of care to home. *Home Healthcare Now*. 2015; 33(3):142-146. doi:10.1097/NHH.0000000000000195.
4. Clark K, Doyle J, Duco S, Lattimer C. *Hot topics in health care: transitions of care: the need for a more effective approach to continuing patient care*. The Joint Commission Resources. <https://www.jointcommission.org/hot_topics_toc/>; 2012 Accessed 20.09.18.
5. Skochelak SE, Hawkins RE, eds. *Value in Health Care*. Philadelphia: Elsevier; 2017 [Chapter 4].

Case 4 answers

4.1: d. Ensuring that the patient's hepatologist and primary care physician are updated with details of the patient's hospitalization
This patient is struggling with abdominal pain, the etiology of which is uncertain, but all imaging studies done to date and her exam and laboratory studies are reassuring. Thus repeating the CT scan would be unlikely to provide any new information. Indeed, imaging overuse is a one

of the largest drivers of medical waste in the United States. Health care professionals must use appropriate care to limit overuse. The framework proposed by the Alliance of Academic Internal Medicine–American College of Physicians has several steps that help clinicians choose a high-value, cost-conscious means of caring for patients: (1) Understand the benefits, harms, and relative costs of the interventions that you are considering. (2) Decrease or eliminate the use of interventions that provide no benefits or may be harmful. (3) Choose interventions and care settings that maximize benefits, minimize harms, and reduce costs. (4) Customize care plans with patients that incorporate their values and address their concerns. (5) Identify system-level opportunities to improve outcomes, minimize harms, and reduce health care waste. Using this framework, repeating the CT scan is more likely to cause harm (radiation exposure) than benefit. Ordering daily laboratory studies is also recognized as another cause of both overuse and waste, and potentially leads to patient harm by causing worsening anemia. Laboratory studies should be ordered judiciously, based on the needs of the individual patient. Opioids are being recognized as a cause of harm to patients, and new guidelines are being put in place to avoid their use for pain control if other medications or modalities can be used. Integration and coordination of care is one of the best ways the clinician can ensure follow-up care and high-value care for this patient. Talking with the patient's primary clinicians may help the hospitalist understand the best way to help this patient address her pain issues without subjecting her to unnecessary testing and medications.

Suggested further readings

1. Cho HJ, Wray CM, Maione S, et al. Right care in hospital medicine: co-creation of ten opportunities in overuse and underuse for improving value in hospital medicine. *J Gen Intern Med*. 2018;33(6):804-806.

2. Esmail L, Wolfson D, Simpson L. *Reducing low value care: research questions identified by researchers, patients, physicians, and stakeholders.* Academy Health. <http://www.academyhealth.org/publications/2016-04/reducing-low-value-care-research-questions-identified-researchers-patients>; 2016 Accessed 20.09.18.
3. Smith CD. Teaching high-value, cost-conscious care to residents: the Alliance for Academic Internal Medicine–American College of Physicians Curriculum. *Ann Intern Med.* 2012;157:284-286.
4. Herzig SJ, Mosher HJ, Calcaterra SL, Jena AB, Nuckols TK. Improving the safety of opioid use for acute noncancer pain in hospitalized adults: a consensus statement from the Society of Hospital Medicine. *J Hosp Med.* 2018;13(4):263-271.

Case 5 answers

Q 5.1: e. Obtain the previous laboratory studies from the primary care provider

This patient is a healthy female, who meets American Society of Anesthesiologists Physical Status (ASA PS) Classification 1 criteria, about to undergo a medium-risk surgery. Multiple studies indicate insufficient evidence for routine testing in healthy individuals unless there are specific clues in the history and physical to warrant testing. A randomized study looking at preoperative testing prior to cataract surgery showed no difference in outcome, regardless of preoperative testing. Any preoperative testing should be based on individual patient characteristics and the surgery to be performed. Nonjudicious use of testing can delay the procedure and lead to further testing to evaluate a clinically insignificant finding. In this case, she reports a history of anemia, but there is no reason to do any testing now since she is asymptomatic. She had tests done 3 months prior, which can be obtained from her primary physician. Patients whose test results in the past 4 months were normal and whose clinical status is stable do not need repeat testing prior to surgery.

A recent study looking at the 2014 health care expenditures for Virginia that would be considered low value showed that low-cost services accounted for 65% of all health care costs and hence led to the largest amount of wasted resources. Low-cost preoperative lab testing for low-risk patients undergoing low-risk surgery accounted for nearly half of unnecessary spending. Thus decreasing waste in health care spending will require the targeted reduction of high-volume, low-value, low-cost services.

Suggested further readings

1. Martin SK, Cifu AS. Routine preoperative laboratory tests for elective surgery. *JAMA.* 2017;318(6):567-568.
2. Cohn SL. Preoperative evaluation for noncardiac surgery. *Ann Intern Med.* 2016;165(6):ITC81-ITC96.
3. Mafi JN, Russell K, Bortz BA, Dachary M, Hazel Jr WA, Fendrick AM. Low-cost, high-volume health services contribute the most to unnecessary health spending. *Health Aff (Millwood).* 2017;36(10):1701-1704.

Case 6 answers

Q 6.1: b. The value of this strategy is likely to be low since the patient stopped smoking last year

The US Preventive Services Task Force recommends annual screening for lung cancer with low-dose CT in adults aged 55 to 80 years who have a 30 pack/year history of smoking and currently smoke or have quit within the past 15 years, based on the results of the National Lung Screening Trial. Although his calculated risk for lung cancer is high, Mr. E's other comorbidities are a competing risk for death and may preclude definitive management if lung cancer is found, which is why screening him for lung cancer would be low value. It has been felt that the highest benefit and hence the highest value of a preventive strategy is when it is applied to the population that it was tested in. Hence choice b would be false. A screening program has to have representation from all disciplines needed to address lung cancer found as a result of screening to be effective and high value. It is likely that screening for lung cancer because of the downstream effects will add to the cost for the US health system, but by providing a meaningful decrease of 20% in lung cancer mortality, it can help improve overall population health.

Suggested further readings

1. Smetana GW, Boiselle PM, Schwartzstein RM. Screening for lung cancer with low-dose computed tomography: grand rounds discussion from the Beth Israel Deaconess Medical Center. *Ann Intern Med.* 2015;162(8):577-582.
2. Guessous I, Cornuz J. Why and how would we implement a lung cancer screening program? *Public Health Rev.* 2015;36:10.

Case 7 answers

Q 7.1: b. Payment reforms to help implement clinical practice improvement initiatives

Understanding the barriers to implementation of Choosing Wisely (CW) recommendations may be required to promote appropriate implementation of this initiative to reduce low-value and unnecessary medical care. Concern regarding medicolegal risk, actual and physician perceived patient requests for tests, and traditional fee-for-service payment models are thought to be key drivers of overutilization of medical services and therefore inadequate use of CW recommendations. Alternatively, payment reforms, which may promote better patient communication and shared decision making, can facilitate wider adaptation of these recommendations. Therefore, choice b is not a potential barrier and the correct answer.

Suggested further readings

1. Zikmund-Fisher BJ, Kullgren JT, Fagerlin A, Klamerus ML, Bernstein SJ, Kerr EA. Perceived barriers to implementing individual Choosing Wisely® recommendations in two national surveys of primary care providers. *J Gen Intern Med.* 2017;32(2):210-217.

2. Colla CH, Mainor AJ. Choosing wisely campaign: valuable for providers who knew about it, but awareness remained constant, 2014–17. *Health Aff (Millwood)*. 2017;36(11):2005-2011.
3. Rich EC. Barriers to Choosing Wisely® in primary care: it's not just about "the money." *J Gen Intern Med*. 2017;32(2):140-142.

Case 8 answers

Q 8.1: c. Assuming copayment assistance programs and coupons resolve financial concerns

Financial burden from medical treatment is increasingly being recognized as a threat to optimal access, quality, and outcomes of care for patients. Providing high-value, true patient-centered care involves not only caring for physical and emotional health, but also for patients' financial well-being. Growing evidence suggests that having a discussion about financial stress or being informed about cost of care may help in lowering distress associated with out-of-pocket cost burden at the patient level. However, physician behaviors, such as not acknowledging or dismissing financial concerns too quickly or reliance on temporary solutions without making long-term plans to reduce spending can lead to loss of an opportunity to provide higher-value care and result in failure of the provider to assess the patient's financial concerns.

Suggested further readings

1. Moriates C, Shah NT, Arora VM. First, do no (financial) harm. *JAMA*. 2013;310(6):577-578.
2. Ubel PA, Zhang CJ, Hesson A, et al. Study of physician and patient communication identifies missed opportunities to help reduce patients' out-of-pocket spending. *Health Aff (Millwood)*. 2016;35(4):654-661.

Q 8.2: d. A 30-year-old male with acute low back pain who has not seen his primary care physician for the last year

Early palliative care defined as "the provision of specialist palliative care services upstream from the end of life, while living with a serious illness" has the potential to improve patient quality of life and satisfaction and decrease symptom burden. It is especially important to consider in patients with life-threatening conditions, extensive comorbidities, and poor psychosocial support. In contrast, the correct answer is a young male who does not have a definitive diagnosis because of not having seen a physician. While he may have needs for pain medication in the short term, a palliative care referral may not be needed at this point in time, unless evaluated by his physician and found to meet any of the above criteria.

Suggested further readings

1. Rabow M, Kvale E, Barbour L, et al. Moving upstream: a review of the evidence of the impact of outpatient palliative care. *J Palliat Med*. 2013;16(12):1540-1549.
2. Davis MP, Temel JS, Balboni T, Glare P. A review of the trials which examine early integration of outpatient and home palliative care for patients with serious illnesses. *Ann Palliat Med*. 2015;4(3):99-121.
3. Temel JS, Greer JA, Muzikansky A, et al. Early palliative care for patients with metastatic non-small-cell lung cancer. *N Engl J Med*. 2010;363(8):733-742.

Q 8.3: a. Helping identify and develop interventions to bend the cost curve for the potentially high-cost patients

Big Data in health care is the extensive health data available from various sources, such as electronic health records (EHRs), medical imaging, genomic sequencing, payer records, pharmaceutical research, wearables, and medical devices. There are abundant opportunities to use this data for improving the quality of care and decreasing costs by being able to track high-cost patients and delivering evidence-based information that can help increase efficiencies. There are still many challenges in the implementation and use of Big Data analytics, such as privacy concerns, quality and accuracy concerns, the possibility of misuse, and unwanted consequences such as restrictive insurance policies, all of which need to be addressed before it can revolutionize the field of health care.

Suggested further readings

1. Bates DW, Saria S, Ohno-Machado L, Shah A, Escobar G. Big Data in health care: using analytics to identify and manage high-risk and high-cost patients. *Health Aff (Millwood)*. 2014;33(7):1123-1131.
2. *NEJM Catalyst*. Healthcare Big Data and the promise of value-based care. <https://catalyst.nejm.org/big-data-healthcare/>; 2018 Accessed 21.09.18.

Case 9 answers

Q 9.1: d. Unnecessary care where eliminating a service would not have changed the quality of care

Medical waste reduces value in health care. Waste in medical care includes many categories, such as excess administration waste, inefficient delivery of services, missed prevention opportunities, medical fraud and abuse, and unnecessary care. Unnecessary care—a service that would have not changed the quality of care—is estimated as the largest category of medical waste, at about one-third of its total cost. In this case, eliminating a cardiac stress would have not provided higher quality care to this patient where the likelihood of uncovering ischemic heart disease would have been extremely rare.

Suggested further readings

1. McGinnis JM, Stuckhardt L, Saunders R, Smith M, eds. *Best Care at Lower Cost: The Path to Continuously Learning Health Care in America*. Washington, DC: National Academies Press; 2013.
2. Mendu ML, McAvay G, Lampert R, Stoehr J, Tinetti ME. Yield of diagnostic tests in evaluating syncopal episodes in older patients. *Arch Intern Med*. 2009;169(14):1299.

Case 10 answers

Q 10.1: d. They are more successful if the implementation strategy includes audit and feedback

EHR-based clinical decision support (CDS) tools can reduce inappropriate test ordering by a moderate amount. Implementing EHR-based CDS tools is associated with greater effectiveness in integrated health care systems. Some studies suggest that audit and feedback strategies are more likely to result in greater effectiveness of CDS tools. Little evidence exists on whether such interventions are associated with harm or unintended consequences. For example, a study of CDS to prevent drug–drug interactions showed it was effective in changing prescribing practices but resulted in delays in treatment for some patients.

Suggested further readings

1. Goldzweig CL, Orshansky G, Paige NM, et al. Electronic health record-based interventions for improving appropriate diagnostic imaging: a systematic review and meta-analysis. *Ann Intern Med.* 2015;162(8):557-565.
2. Gupta A, Ip IK, Raja AS, Andruchow JE, Sodickson A, Khorasani R. Effect of clinical decision support on documented guideline adherence for head CT in emergency department patients with mild traumatic brain injury. *J Am Med Inform Assoc.* 2014;21(2):E347-E351.

Case 11 answers

Q 11.1: b. Limiting your intervention to target poorly controlled type 2 diabetes mellitus patients to maximize the value of your intervention

In managing chronic diseases in general, effectively targeting high-risk populations will be important to achieving maximum value. Several researchers suggest that the magnitude of improvement in diabetes-related outcomes, including savings, may be associated with the risk status of the target population. The type of the intervention is also critical for better outcomes. Often single facet interventions are less effective. For example, team-based interventions were shown to be more effective than nurse-based approaches, and both team- and nurse-based approaches were more effective than programs designed merely to improve patient management.

Suggested further reading

1. McKethan A, Shepard M, Kocot SL, et al. *Improving quality and value in the U.S. health care system.* Bipartisan Policy Center. <https://bipartisanpolicy.org/wp-content/uploads/sites/default/files/BPC8-09-PCHC%20Qual%20rpt-8-20-09.pdf>; 2009 Accessed 21.09.18.

Case 12 answers

Q 12.1: d. The evidence suggests that the association between health care cost and quality is poorly understood

According to a systematic review by Hussey et al., the magnitude and the direction of relationship between quality and cost is poorly understood, mainly because of different ways published studies measured cost and quality.

Suggested further reading

1. Hussey PS, Wertheimer S, Mehrotra A. The association between health care quality and cost: a systematic review. *Ann Intern Med.* 2013;158(1):27-34.

Case 13 answers

Q 13.1: a. Patient experience of care

In a national survey of Medicare Part C patients between 2006 and 2012, African Americans and Latinos often report care experiences similar with those of non-Latino whites. Significant disparities by race and ethnicity are seen in quality of care for chronic disease control and use of behavioral health services, including mental and substance use disorder treatment. Preventive care services are closely linked to access to primary care services, which are often less accessible for minorities and low-income populations.

Suggested further reading

1. Fiscella K, Sanders MR. Racial and ethnic disparities in the quality of health care. *Annu Rev Public Health.* 2016;37: 375-394.

Case 14 answers

Q 14.1: c. Patients treated with a chemotherapy regimen of docetaxel-5FU-cisplatin (TPF) showed a greater response of metastatic lesions compared to patients treated with other chemotherapy regimens

A patient's utility functions represent his or her preferences of trade-offs. This may include cost and the likelihood of a cure, but for many conditions it also includes the level of tolerance for physical side effects or psychosocial impact on daily life. Health-related quality of life (HRQoL) outcomes can be helpful as prognostic guides to aid in medical decision making. Choice c describes a clinical outcome that answers an evidence-based medicine (EBM)–PICO (Problem/Patient/Population, Intervention/Indicator, Comparison, Outcome) question but does not incorporate patient values. Choices a, b, and d each have a patient symptom outcome (swallowing, dry mouth, and pain) that may be an important utility function for patients to consider. For some patients one or more of these symptoms may be important enough to forgo treatment if the likelihood of symptoms were high. Studies are increasingly including HRQoL assessments. Stratifying patients by their baseline HRQoL in future studies will provide further guidance in decision making with regard to overall well-being in addition to clinical response to treatment. HRQoL assessments can play an important role in achieving the goals of the personalized medicine movement by taking into account patient preferences (utility) and biologic variables.

Suggested further readings

1. Licitra L, Mesía R, Keilholz U. Individualised quality of life as a measure to guide treatment choices in squamous cell carcinoma of the head and neck. *Oral Oncol.* 2016;52:18-23.

2. Guenne C, Fayette J, Cosmidis A, et al. Curative treatment can be an option for patients with metastatic squamous cell cancer of the head and neck. *Drug Des Devel Ther.* 2014;8:2549-2553.

Case 15 answers

Q 15.1: c. "What have your other patients who have my condition chosen for treatment?"

Value-based medicine relates the costs of an intervention to the value placed on the result of the intervention. This is often calculated in cost per quality adjusted life year. In determining the value of an intervention, a variety of instruments may be used to assess the patient's preferences. One common analysis calculates the time (years of remaining life) that someone would consider giving up to gain a particular outcome. Choice a may demonstrate a desired optimism, but she does not express a weighting of what she would be willing to gain for a shortened life. She is delegating that to the physician and this statement is, therefore, not an important patient value assessment. In choice d, though also delegating the value assessment to the physician, the patient is asking the physician to be her proxy. Studies have shown that nearly 90% of the time people underestimate the reduction in quality of life caused by the disease. Relying then on the surrogate's opinion is a poor approximation of the patient's value. Studies that help to inform patients on quality of life outcomes must be standardized to match the patient's condition. A comparison of a similar treatment for a different condition (diabetes versus macular degeneration) will not accurately inform the patient of the potential quality of life impact. Knowing what others with the same condition have chosen demonstrates the patient is assessing how the preferences of others might be in alignment with her own.

Suggested further reading

1. Brown MM, Brown GC. Update on value-based medicine. *Curr Opin Ophthalmol.* 2013;24(3):183-189.

Case 16 answers

Q 16.1: b. Review of the records from her hospital of all 40-year-old men with pulmonary embolism

Performing unnecessary tests affects patient care negatively in several ways. Exposing patients to radiation unnecessarily may increase the risk of developing other cancers. From a value perspective, there are considerations both at the patient level and at the system level. The increased cost associated with ordering unnecessary tests creates very little value for the patient, other than the reassurance of a normal exam. That value will vary inversely to the cost of the testing. Benchmarking and use of probability tools can help to inform whether testing patterns are appropriate for the population being evaluated.

Choice b will not inform the pretest probability that a CTPA will provide a sufficient posttest probability that pulmonary embolism is present. It will provide a retrospective view of patients with the diagnosis of this condition and can help to define the characteristics of 40-year-olds who have had it, but is not useful at helping to inform the

incidence of pulmonary embolism in the population. The latter is a necessary attribute to help with the pretest calculations. Choice a would inform not only the incidence of pulmonary embolism in the community but also provide for a view of the potential variations in providers' thresholds for ordering CTPAs and is an important step in any process improvement project. Choices c and d will provide for understanding and implementation of tools that utilize pretest probability to inform the likelihood that a particular test will be useful in the diagnostic workup.

Suggested further readings

1. Osman M, Subedi SK, Ahmed A, et al. Computed tomography pulmonary angiography is overused to diagnose pulmonary embolism in the emergency department of academic community hospital. *J Community Hosp Intern Med Perspect.* 2018;8(1):6-10.
2. Raja AS, Ip IK, Prevedello LM, et al. Effect of computerized clinical decision support on the use and yield of CT pulmonary angiography in the emergency department. *Radiology.* 2012;262(2):468-474.

Q 16.2: d. Outcome bias

Outcome bias is defined by allowing a prior event or decision outcome to influence subsequent independent decisions. This best fits the scenario of missing a pulmonary embolism in a young patient recently, even though the current case independently has a low probability of the condition.

Availability bias defines scenarios where the estimation or probability of an event is influenced by the ease with which previous events can be brought to mind. This would best fit scenarios where physicians feel they have seen this clinical presentation many times, and they do not assess the current patient's risks independently.

Anchoring bias describes scenarios where the diagnosis is suggested and then accepted rather than other alternatives being considered. An example would be if Mr. F was referred to the emergency department by his primary care physician because of concern for a pulmonary embolism. Despite a low-probability Wells score, the emergency department physician could let the primary care physician's concern carry greater weight in her decision making.

Optimism bias occurs when there is a favorable expectation for an outcome even when the situation may dictate otherwise. This would be the opposite scenario to this case where a CTPA was not ordered, despite an intermediate-risk Wells score because the emergency department physician felt the patient was too young to have a pulmonary embolism.

Suggested further readings

1. Brush JE. Decision-making shortcuts: the good and the bad. <https://knowledgeplus.nejm.org/blog/decision-making-shortcuts-good-bad/>; 2015 Accessed 21.09.18.
2. Blumenthal-Barby JS, Krieger H. Cognitive biases and heuristics in medical decision making: a critical review using a systematic search strategy. *Med Decis Making.* 2015;35(4):539-557.

Case 17 answers

Q 17.1: d. Utilize principles of time-driven, activity-based costing (TDABC) that you have seen in recent articles

Though each of these may be helpful in improving the value/cost equation, the principles of TDABC are felt to be the most comprehensive, taking into account the cost of each component of an activity. This includes personnel time and facility costs as well as component costs of the procedure or visit.

TDABC was developed by Kaplan and Anderson at Harvard Business School. It utilizes the unit cost as well as the time taken to perform the activity to estimate the total costs of an activity. TDABC may provide more thorough estimates of efficiency and cost details than traditional costing methods. On the other hand, TDABC is time consuming and often costly, which may explain why health care entities have been slow to adopt this methodology.

The other interventions are more limited in scope. SOAP-V has been demonstrated to provide medical students with a framework to feel more comfortable in discussing the cost of an intervention on the value to the patient and the cost to the health care system as a whole. Studies have shown that diabetics with hemoglobin A1c values greater than 8 have higher postoperative costs, though it is not clear that postponing surgery leads to cost savings or increases value to the patient.

Suggested further readings

1. Kaplan RS, Anderson SR. Time-driven activity-based costing. *Harv Bus Rev.* 2004;82:131-138.
2. Mercier G, Naro G. Costing hospital surgery services: the method matters. *PLoS One.* 2014;9(5):E97290. doi:10.1371/journal.pone.0097290.
3. Moser EM, Huang GC, Packer CD, et al. SOAP-V: Introducing a method to empower medical students to be change agents in bending the cost curve. *J Hosp Med.* 2016;3:217-220.
4. Keel G, Savage C, Rafiq M, Mazzocato P. Time-driven activity-based costing in health care: a systematic review of the literature. *Health Policy.* 2017;121(7):755-763.
5. Chen A, Sabharwal S, Akhtar K, Makaram N, Gupte CM. Time-driven activity based costing of total knee replacement surgery at a London teaching hospital. *Knee.* 2015:22(6):640-645.
6. Harris AH, Bowe TR, Gupta S, Ellerbe LS, Giori NJ. Hemoglobin A1C as a marker for surgical risk in diabetic patients undergoing total joint arthroplasty. *J Arthroplasty.* 2103;28(suppl 8):S25-S29.
7. McLawhorn AS, Southren D, Wang YC, Marx RG, Dodwell ER. Cost-effectiveness of bariatric surgery prior to total knee arthroplasty in the morbidly obese: a computer model-based evaluation. *J Bone Joint Surg Am.* 2016;98(2):E6.

Case 18 answers

Q 18.1: b. False

Every treatment decision may have a financial impact on the patient's financial well-being, in addition to her health. Helping patients navigate the trade-offs related to out-of-pocket costs, physicians should work to ensure that their patients achieve the best outcome. Helping this patient understand how low-value care is determined may be helpful to allow her to distinguish appropriate from inappropriate care. In addition, an open discussion with the patient to understand potential concerns will help prevent the wrong assumptions that a copayment will be a barrier for selecting a test. Charlesworth and colleagues have reported a lack of an association between care delivered and insurance type.

Suggested further readings

1. Chalmers K, Badgery-Parker T, Pearson SA, Brett J, Scott IA, Elshaug AG. Developing indicators for measuring low-value care: mapping Choosing Wisely recommendations to hospital data. *BMC Res Notes.* 2018;11:163.
2. Charlesworth CJ, Meath TH, Schwartz AL, McConnell KJ. Comparison of low-value care in Medicaid vs commercially insured populations. *JAMA Intern Med.* 2016;176(7):998-1004.
3. Riggs KR, Ubel PA. Overcoming barriers to discussing out-of-pocket costs with patients. *JAMA Intern Med.* 2014;174(6):849-850.

7

Patient Safety

Tamala S. Bradham, PhD, DHA, CPPS, CPHQ, Kendra Parekh, MD

Cases and questions

Case 1

Mrs. Susan Smith is a 56-year-old African American female patient admitted to the hospital with complaints of substernal chest pain and numbness in her left arm. She has a prior history of high cholesterol and a 50-pack/year history of smoking. She is admitted to the observation unit where a technician draws cardiac enzymes and a nurse performs an electrocardiogram. A few hours later, the physician on call is reviewing Mrs. Smith's chart and discovers that the labs in her electronic health record (EHR) are not hers. Upon discussion with the technician and the nurse, it is discovered that the labs were labeled by a distracted technician with the patient's roommate's name: Mrs. Sarah Smith.

Q 1.1: What is the best way to classify the error described in this scenario?
a. Preventable adverse event
b. Negligent adverse event
c. Near miss
d. Malpractice

Q 1.2: In talking to the team, the physician discovers that this has happened before with other patients who have similar names. Which of the following attributes is most characteristic of this type of occurrence?
a. Preventable
b. Nonpreventable
c. Negligent
d. None of the above

Q 1.3: Which category best fits this type of occurrence?
a. Memory lapse
b. Attention failure

c. Knowledge error
d. Cognitive error

Q 1.4: The physician is concerned that this type of problem might happen again and decides to undertake a project to reduce that possibility. Which of the following is the best tool or strategy to employ?
a. Counseling the employees involved about their behavior
b. Use of an SBAR tool
c. A mandatory event reporting system
d. A voluntary event reporting system

Case 2

Multiple traumas are sent to a local hospital following a motor vehicle accident. One patient, Mr. Smith, is evaluated in the emergency department and taken immediately to surgery. Once stabilized, he is transferred to the intensive care unit (ICU) during shift change. The bedside nurse administers intravenous (IV) insulin (a high-alert medication) to treat a severely elevated potassium, per physician's orders. The hospital policy requires that the medication barcode and the patient identification (ID) band be scanned into the EHR prior to medication administration. The nurse does not scan the barcode or ID band because the scanner is often unavailable or broken. The incorrect patient receives the medication, and that patient suffers a severe episode of low blood glucose producing altered mental status that rapidly resolves with correct treatment. There are no long-term sequelae.

Q 2.1: What is the best way to classify the error described in this scenario?
a. Preventable adverse event
b. Negligent adverse event
c. Near miss
d. Malpractice

Q 2.2: What is the best way to classify the nurse's intent in this scenario?
a. Violation
b. Slip
c. Lapse
d. Mistake

Q 2.3: The quality improvement office investigates this event and learns that overriding the scanning of the medication barcode is considered a common practice for that unit. Which of the following best describes this practice?
a. Just Culture
b. Flattening the hierarchy
c. Regression to the mean
d. Normalization of deviance

Q 2.4: There were several failures associated with this event. Which of the following choices would be considered the primary active failure?
a. Admission to the floor during shift change
b. Identification of the patient
c. Overriding the medication scanning requirement
d. Administering the medication to the wrong patient

Q 2.5: What next step should the medical patient safety adviser take to reduce this type of error in the future?
a. Complete a risk assessment
b. Question the nurse who made the error
c. Wait to do any formal review and watch for trends of this type of event
d. Conduct an event analysis with a process map

Case 3

A patient was recently hospitalized and started on an increased dose of blood pressure medication. The patient is being seen in follow-up with his primary care physician. At the conclusion of the visit, the physician instructs the patient to go to the lab for bloodwork to monitor for side effects of the increased dosage. The patient is busy after the visit and does not go for bloodwork. Several days pass, and the physician notes that the bloodwork has not been completed. The physician made a note in the EHR that the patient needs to be called but forgot to forward the note to an office staff member for follow-up. The labs never got drawn. The patient ends up in the emergency department with an electrolyte abnormality and mild kidney injury due to the medication.

Q 3.1: What is the best way to classify the error described in this scenario?
a. Preventable adverse event
b. Negligent adverse event
c. Near miss
d. Malpractice

Q 3.2: What is the best way to classify the physician's intent in this scenario?
a. Lapse
b. Mistake
c. Slip
d. Violation

Q 3.3: Which category best fits this type of occurrence?
a. Memory lapse
b. Attention failure
c. Knowledge error
d. Cognitive error

Q 3.4: The physician discusses the event with colleagues in the practice. The group would like to explore latent and active failures in this case. Which of the following would be the most appropriate next step?
a. Explore active failures by analyzing the structure of the office staff
b. Explore active failures by investigating the process of physician notification for missed lab appointments
c. Explore latent failures by investigating communication processes between physicians and office staff in the EHR
d. Explore latent failures by reviewing the involved physician's charts in detail to determine the number of similar occurrences

Case 4

The Agency for Healthcare Research and Quality (AHRQ) Hospital Survey on Patient Safety Culture reported that Grand Hospital has an "excellent" patient safety grade. Due to this, the administration developed a new strategic plan to promote a Just Culture at Grand Hospital.

Q 4.1: Identify the best strategy that should be included in the strategic plan for the employees at Grand Hospital.
a. Develop and implement a second victim program
b. Revise current patient safety event policy to include that any person(s) involved in a patient safety event resulting in harm to the patient will be placed on a mandatory 30-day administrative leave immediately following the reporting of the event
c. Develop and implement a mandatory oral presentation of the patient safety event during the mortality, morbidity, and improvement conferences
d. Eliminate anonymous reporting of safety events

Q 4.2: Identify the best strategy for disclosing an adverse event due to a medical error that should be included in the strategic plan at Grand Hospital.
a. A patient safety office/risk management office will provide an explanation of why the error occurred and how their health care providers were able to minimize the impact to the patient, apologize to the patient, and provide an overview on how Grand Hospital will review the error that occurred, to minimize it from happening again to another patient
b. A Grand Hospital administrator or chief of staff will provide an explanation of why the error occurred, apologize to the patient, and explain how Grand Hospital will take actions to minimize the chance of this occurring to another patient
c. Health care providers will provide an explanation of why the error occurred and how they were able to minimize the impact to the patient, apologize to the patient, and provide an overview on how Grand Hospital will thoroughly review the error that occurred, to minimize it from happening again to another patient

d. A patient liaison will provide an explanation of why the error occurred and how their health care providers were able to minimize the impact to the patient, apologize to the patient, and provide an overview on how Grand Hospital will review the error that occurred, to minimize it from happening again to another patient.

Case 5

There are several different types of errors. For the following examples, identify the type of error.

Q 5.1: Missed diagnosis due to a misread computed tomography (CT) scan
a. Faulty knowledge
b. Faulty data gathering
c. Faulty synthesis information processing or verification
d. Faulty communication

Q 5.2: Delayed diagnosis of breast cancer due to failure of a practitioner to obtain a screening mammogram
a. Faulty knowledge
b. Faulty data gathering
c. Faulty synthesis information processing or verification
d. Faulty communication

Q 5.3: A patient with nausea, vomiting, and diarrhea is diagnosed with gastroenteritis but later found to have appendicitis.
a. Faulty knowledge
b. Faulty data gathering
c. Faulty synthesis information processing or verification
d. Faulty communication

Case 6

Bias comes in many different forms. For the following questions, identify the type of bias described in each scenario.

Q 6.1: A medical student just learned about aortic dissection. That afternoon they see a patient in clinic with chest pain and prioritize aortic dissection first on the differential diagnosis.
a. Omission bias
b. Hindsight bias
c. Availability bias
d. Search-satisfying error

Q 6.2: A mother accompanies her 2-year-old son to the pediatrician's office and expresses concerns about her son's delay in learning to talk, ignoring her when she calls him, and not startling at loud noises. The pediatrician refers the child for a speech-language evaluation, and the child starts speech and language services. A year later, the child still has minimal speech and language. At the encouragement of the speech-language pathologist, the pediatrician orders a hearing evaluation. The boy has bilateral moderate to severe sensorineural hearing loss.
a. Anchoring bias
b. Commission bias
c. Regret bias
d. Availability bias

Q 6.3: A 55-year-old male patient with alcoholism and a history of pancreatitis presents with severe midepigastric abdominal pain and shortness of breath after several days of drinking. The physician thinks this is pancreatitis and obtains a lipase. The physician does not order an electrocardiogram (ECG). The lipase returns as normal, and the subsequent ECG demonstrates an acute heart attack.
a. Commission bias
b. Confirmation bias
c. Aggregate bias
d. Regret bias

Q 6.4: A radiologist reads a chest X-ray of a patient with a fever and cough as having a lobar pneumonia but fails to notice an enlarging lung nodule.
a. Sunk-cost effect/bias
b. Hindsight bias
c. Omission bias
d. Search-satisfying error

Case 7

The most common reason for a paid malpractice claim in the ambulatory setting is a result of a diagnostic error. In the 2015 Institute of Medicine report, "Improving Diagnosis in Healthcare," eight goals were outlined to reduce this common error.

Q 7.1: From the following list, which one was NOT included as one of the eight goals?
a. Teamwork
b. Health information technologies (HIT)
c. Partnering with patients and their families
d. Payment for services are denied that are a result of a diagnostic error

Q 7.2: Which of the following is an example of malpractice?
a. The physician orders an antibiotic. The patient suffers a severe allergic reaction and requires admission to the intensive care unit
b. A patient is undergoing general anesthesia for a surgical procedure and has a heart attack. The patient is no longer able to work in his job due to this medical condition
c. A patient has a total knee replacement and does not participate in therapy as recommended. Subsequently, the patient falls and requires revision surgery
d. A surgeon uses an incorrectly sterilized instrument during a surgery. The patient subsequently develops a severe bacterial infection and dies

Case 8

An event analysis is being conducted on a potential handover communication event that led to a prolonged length of stay and permanent serious harm to the patient. The patient safety team and risk management learned about the event through an anonymous, voluntary report of the event. The managers and supervisors were interviewed to determine who was directly involved with the event and a meeting time was scheduled.

Q 8.1: The medical patient safety officer is facilitating the discussion with the individuals involved in the event. To ensure active dialogue among the people involved, what should the facilitator do first when starting the meeting?
a. Have everyone introduce themselves and their role in patient care and then provide the purpose and ground rules for the meeting
b. Provide the purpose and ground rules for the meeting and present the process flow map and respectfully ask questions about each item
c. Have everyone introduce themselves and provide the action plan after receiving input from the individuals
d. Provide the purpose and ground rules for the meeting and present factual data collected from multiple sources about the event

Q 8.2: During the action planning process, the facilitator wants to promote a Just Culture. What is something the facilitator can do to support this goal?
a. For each action item, assign a person to be responsible for ensuring that it is completed
b. Mitigate negative statements about an individual involved and remind people to use titles, not names
c. Develop a 30-, 60-, 90-day report by the managers of the individuals involved in the event
d. Ask for a volunteer to share the information learned from the event analysis at an upcoming mortality, morbidity, and improvement conference

Answers

Case 1 answers

Q 1.1: c. Near miss
This is an example of a near miss. The patient did not suffer harm, and the problem was identified at a point when its downstream consequences could be prevented. This is not an adverse event because no harm occurred to the patient. While this could be considered an error, meaning the planned action was not completed because the laboratory specimen was drawn but from the wrong patient, it is not the best answer. Because no injury occurred, the event does not meet the definition of malpractice.

Q 1.2: a. Preventable
This near miss is preventable. The question states that this has happened before, and one might reasonably anticipate that two patients with similar names located in the same room might be at high risk for errors. Because the event could have been anticipated, it would be incorrect to describe the error as nonpreventable. Negligence is defined as when a person fails to exercise the care typically expected by a careful person in the same scenario. For an event to be categorized as malpractice, negligence must be established.

Q 1.3: b. Attention failure
This event could best be characterized as an attention failure because the case points out that the technician was distracted. A memory lapse may have also occurred, but this is not the best answer. A knowledge error occurs

when there is a gap in understanding of how to handle an issue. A cognitive error occurs when there is an unconscious mistake. These types of failures are shown in Fig. 7.1.

Q 1.4: d. A voluntary event reporting system
Of those listed, the best strategy would be to implement a voluntary reporting system so one could begin to understand the scope and nature of these types of events. When implementing a reporting system, one must balance the workload on the end user with the benefits provided by the system. Implementation of a mandatory reporting system for low-level errors would be difficult, given the potential burden placed on health care workers. While having a conversation with the employees involved in the event might be appropriate, counseling them about their behavior would not. Use of an SBAR tool (i.e., a communication tool often used during care transitions: Situation, Background, Assessment, Recommendation) or a checklist would not likely solve the underlying problems described in the case.

Case 2 answers

Q 2.1: b. Negligent adverse event
This event is best classified as a negligent adverse event because the standard of care was violated when the nurse did not follow the hospital policy to scan the medication barcode and ID band prior to administering a high-alert medication. The patient subsequently suffered harm (low blood glucose and altered mental status). A preventable adverse event is considered an adverse event that is avoidable and is considered attributable to the error. While this event could have been prevented by following hospital protocols, the error occurred due to the nurse violating protocol (not scanning the barcodes) and is considered to be negligent. The event is not a near miss because the event reached the patient as evidenced by the low blood glucose and altered mental status. Although there was evidence of injury (low blood glucose and altered mental status), there were no lasting damages. Thus malpractice is not the best choice for this question.

Q 2.2: a. Violation
When evaluating the intent when an error occurs, it is best to ask these three questions: (1) Was the action intentional? (2) Did the action occur as planned? (3) Did the action bring about the expected outcomes? In this scenario, the nurse's action was intentional (purposely bypassed the policy on scanning the patient and medication) but did not occur as planned (the wrong patient received the medication) and did not result in an expected outcome (the patient had an adverse reaction to the medication administered). Based on this, we would classify the nurse's intent as a violation. While the action did not occur as planned, this is not considered a slip because the nurse did not purposely give the wrong patient the medication. This is not considered a lapse because the nurse did not forget to scan the patient or medication; the nurse made the choice not to scan the barcodes because the equipment is often not available or broken. This would not be classified as a mistake. A mistake

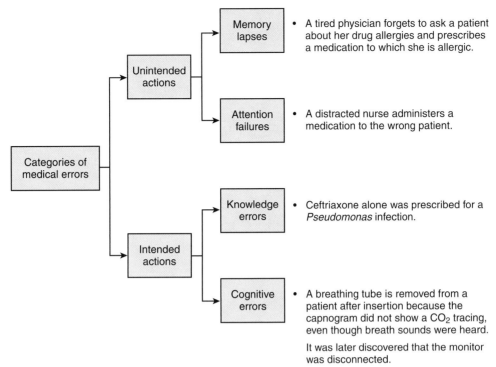

Fig. 7.1 Attention Failure Chart (Lawson LE, Ehrenfeld JM, Walsh D. Patient safety. In: Skochelak SE, Hawkins RE, Lawson LE, Starr SR, Borkan JM, Gonzalo JD, eds. *Health Systems Science*. Philadelphia: Elsevier; 2016:55.)

occurs when someone does something thought to be correct but was not. The nurse knew the barcodes needed to be scanned but chose not to follow the policy thereby bypassing an important safeguard.

Q 2.3: d. Normalization of deviance

The correct answer is normalization of deviance. When the quality improvement officer investigated this event, he spoke to several people on that unit and learned that it was common practice to not use the scanners. By interviewing multiple people with similar credentials on the same unit, he was able to determine that this was more of an environmental issue than an isolated, individual incident. This is a common methodology in patient safety, called the substitution test. The substitution test is used to determine if normalization of deviance has occurred. In the substitution test you ask at least three individuals with similar backgrounds and training and in a similar situation and environment if they would act in a similar manner to the individual being evaluated. If the three people answer "yes," then the problem is not the individual but the environment in which they work. If any of the people interviewed answer "no," then it is more likely that the individual is responsible for the error. When we take shortcuts that deviate from protocols, accept lower standards, or conform to a different level of expectation, then a new normal is created. When people drift from standards and policies without resistance or questioning, then this is referred to as normalization of deviance. Just Culture is not correct because this is when every employee advocates for an environment where safety concerns can be addressed in a nonpunitive manner. This does not appear to be a flattening the hierarchy

scenario, which is where all members of the team feel safe in providing input, are valued for advocating for safety concerns, and are not criticized for doing so. Research suggests that near misses occur 3 to 300 times more often than adverse events, thus flattening the hierarchy is one such strategy to encourage reporting. Finally, regression to the mean is not correct since this is a statistical phenomenon that often leads to inaccurate conclusions regarding the effects of the intervention provided when you have outliers or skewed data.

Q 2.4: b. Identification of the patient

While there were multiple issues in this scenario, it is important to identify the potential failures that occurred in the "Swiss cheese" model, to develop an action plan to mitigate future harm. Considering that all four of these issues occurred, identifying the primary active error will help guide the conversation around identifying process improvements to the system. When starting to engage with any patient, the first thing anyone does is confirm that he or she has the correct patient. Health professionals must ensure they have the right patient before conducting a history interview, performing an examination, or developing a treatment plan. Thus identification of the patient is the correct response for this question. Admission to the floor during shift change, which is highly dissatisfying for nurses who are about to leave after a long shift, is not the primary active failure. While the remaining two choices are considered active errors—overriding the medication scanning requirement and administering the medication to the wrong patient—they are not the primary failures. The nurse could have the correct medication for the patient matching her electronic medication system but would not know she has the incorrect patient without scanning the patient ID or asking the patient first. By scanning the patient first or confirming patient identification in another policy-approved manner, the nurse would have discovered that she did not have the correct patient, the correct EHR displayed on the computer, and/or the correct medication, and would not administer the medication.

Q 2.5: d. Conduct an event analysis with a process map

Once determined that an adverse event occurred, the medical patient safety adviser would want to conduct an event analysis, or a root cause analysis, with a process map to learn about what happened and how to prevent this type of error in the future. Completing a risk assessment is also an important component in the prevention of medical errors and adverse events, but these are often completed by the risk management officers and are often in parallel to the patient safety advisers. While the manager or charge nurse may ask the bedside nurse about the event, the medical patient safety adviser will not question the nurse outside the peer-protected meeting. Since the error resulted in harm to the patient, the medical patient safety officer will want to conduct an event analysis instead of waiting for this type of error to occur again. If the event would have been a near miss and not normal practice for that unit, then the medical patient safety officer might have continued to monitor overall reporting trends.

Case 3 answers

Q 3.1: a. Preventable adverse event

This error is best classified as a preventable adverse event because there was a failure of a planned action to be completed as intended (having the nurse notify the patient to get lab work completed) and the patient suffered an adverse event (electrolyte abnormality and mild kidney injury). This error is not a negligent adverse event because the legal definition of negligence is not met and the standard of care was not violated. This error is not classified as a near miss because the patient suffered harm as evidenced by the electrolyte abnormality and mild kidney injury. This error is not an example of malpractice because a negligent adverse event did not occur.

Q 3.2: a. Lapse

When examining errors, the level of intent of the practitioner's action can be analyzed to help understand the nature of the error. This case represents a lapse because the physician missed that the message did not get sent to the nurse as intended and he forgot to follow up with the nurse. A mistake occurs if a practitioner does something that he or she thought was correct but was not. In this case, the physician's actions were correct, but it was the failure of the physician to send the message to the nurse and to follow up that resulted in the error. A slip occurs when an action does not occur as planned. In this case, the physician did not perform the intended action. A violation occurs when an action is deliberate or illegal. In this scenario, the physician was trying to follow up

with the patient to ensure that the correct labs were completed.

Q 3.3: a. Memory lapse

There are multiple classification systems for medical errors. One system classifies medical errors into intended and unintended actions. In the scenario, the error is best classified as a memory lapse because the physician forgot to forward the message to office personnel. There is nothing in the scenario that indicates the physician was distracted while working in the office, so attention failure is not the best categorization. Knowledge and cognitive errors are intended actions. A knowledge error occurs when there is inaccurate or insufficient knowledge. The physician knew that the patient needed the laboratory studies but forgot to ensure that the message was appropriately sent to the nurse. Thus this is not a knowledge error. Similarly, a cognitive error would occur if an incorrect decision were made or information was synthesized inappropriately. In this scenario, the physician knew what needed to be done but forgot to ensure the message about lab work was sent to the nurse.

Q 3.4: c. Explore latent failures by investigating communication processes between physicians and office staff in the EHR

Reason discussed a persons' approach and a systems' approach to error. The persons' approach focuses on errors of individuals directly providing care at the bedside. These individuals are referred to as the "sharp end." Failures at the sharp end are considered *active failures*. The systems' approach assumes that human error will occur and that systems surrounding the caregivers must be designed to prevent/minimize error. The "blunt end" refers to the systems and processes that are removed from patient contact but still influence patient care. Failures at the blunt end are considered *latent failures*. The best response from the physician group would thus be to explore latent failures by looking at the communication process between physicians and nurses in the EHR. For choice a, the structure of the office staff is at the blunt end and thus not an active failure. Similarly, for choice b, the process of physician notification is at the blunt end and thus not an active failure. For choice d, reviewing the involved physician's charts is focusing on the sharp end and the direct care that the physician provided. This would be an active, not a latent, failure.

Case 4 answers

Q 4.1: a. Develop and implement a second victim program

Making any change takes time. Trying to foster a Just Culture is no exception. With an excellent patient safety grade, as determined by the AHRQ survey, Grand Hospital employees seem to have embraced a culture of safety. Moving toward a Just Culture, however, requires that the entire institution thoroughly evaluate all circumstances and mitigating factors associated with patient safety events with a keen understanding of the processes employed for improvement before assigning any blame to individuals. When establishing a Just Culture, AHRQ promotes three actions: building awareness, implementing policies that support a Just Culture, and building Just Culture principles into practices and all aspects of daily work. It is evident that Grand Hospital employees are aware of the importance of patient safety and reporting safety events. When reviewing their policies, it will be important to clearly define how Grand Hospital will apply Reason's Just Culture model by distinguishing the difference between inadvertent human error and egregious disregard to safety. While placing an individual on administrative leave may seem helpful, it is actually counterproductive in a Just Culture. The involved individual would most likely feel personally attacked and blamed, and the level of harm to the patient may range from mild (e.g., skinned knee from a fall) to severe or even death. It is likely that many factors contributing to the harm would be beyond any one individual. Requiring individuals to speak in front of colleagues may also be perceived as a punishment and may subject them to uncomfortable questions that they may not be ready to share. Eliminating anonymous reporting of safety events has been shown to result in fewer events being reported and an increase in adverse safety events. The next step in Grand Hospital's journey of establishing a Just Culture would be to develop and implement a second victim program. When adverse outcomes occur, even when it is a known complication or risk, health care professionals are impacted, and this can lead to the providers feeling shame and humiliation, isolating themselves from colleagues, or fearing punishment. Second victim programs can help minimize burnout and mental health issues that are often associated with how the institution managed the situation and provides support to employees.

Q 4.2: c. Health care providers will provide an explanation of why the error occurred and how they were able to minimize the impact to the patient, apologize to the patient, and provide an overview on how Grand Hospital will thoroughly review the error that occurred, to minimize it from happening again to another patient

The best strategy for disclosing an adverse event due to a medical error is for the health care professional to provide an explanation of why the error occurred and how the impact to the patient was minimized, apologize to the patient, and provide an overview on how the hospital will ensure the error does not occur again. While it is helpful for the health care professional to consult with the patient safety office or risk management office, neither the patient safety office, the risk management office, the hospital administrator, or a patient liaison should be the first person to discuss the error with the patient and/or the patient's family. The patient and family may have questions that only the health care professional can answer. Furthermore, patients who feel like they can have open, honest conversations with their health care team are more likely to continue their relationship even after a medical error.

Case 5 answers

Q 5.1: a. Faulty knowledge

While efforts are made to learn how the system contributed to the patient safety event and/or medical error, health care providers will also continue to make errors. Evaluation of systems and processes for opportunities to improve safety is easier than evaluating the human components to errors. Cognitive science is the study of the human

components and how decisions are made. A missed diagnosis due to a misread CT scan represents a cognitive contribution to error. Specifically, this example represents faulty knowledge due to insufficient diagnostic skill. While faulty data gathering is an example of a cognitive contribution to error, examples of faulty data gathering would be ineffective or incomplete history and physical or failure to screen. A misread CT scan does not represent faulty data gathering. Faulty synthesis of information processing or verification is an example of a cognitive contribution to error, but a misread CT scan is not an example of this. Examples of faulty synthesis of information processing or verification would be overapplication of a "rule of thumb" or drawing an incorrect conclusion from a correct test result. While communication is essential in a patient safety culture, faulty communication is not a cognitive contribution to error.

Q 5.2: b. Faulty data gathering

A delayed diagnosis of breast cancer due to the failure of a provider to obtain a screening mammogram represents a cognitive contribution to error. Specifically, this example represents faulty data gathering due to the failure to appropriately screen. The correct data—a screening mammogram—was not obtained and the patient suffered harm. While faulty knowledge is an example of a cognitive contribution to error, examples of faulty knowledge would include inadequate or defective knowledge, diagnostic skills, or therapeutic skills. Faulty synthesis of information processing or verification is an example of a cognitive contribution to error, but failure to screen is not an example of this. Examples of faulty synthesis of information processing or verification would be overapplication of a "rule of thumb" or drawing an incorrect conclusion from a correct test result. While communication is essential in a patient safety culture, faulty communication is not a cognitive contribution to error.

Q 5.3: c. Faulty synthesis information processing or verification

A patient with nausea, vomiting, and diarrhea diagnosed with gastroenteritis and later found to have appendicitis is an example of a cognitive contribution to error. This example demonstrates faulty synthesis of information processing or verification. Specifically, it represents a failed heuristic where the practitioner assumed gastroenteritis given the presence of nausea, vomiting, and diarrhea and failed to consider alternative diagnoses. While faulty knowledge is an example of a cognitive contribution to error, examples of faulty knowledge would include inadequate or defective knowledge, diagnostic skills, or therapeutic skills. Faulty data gathering is another example of a cognitive contribution to error, examples of faulty data gathering would be ineffective or incomplete history and physical or failure to screen. While communication is essential in a patient safety culture, faulty communication is not a cognitive contribution to error.

Case 6 answers

Q 6.1: c. Availability bias

Intuition is a key skill for predicting when a patient is critically ill or what complication may occur, especially when time is of the essence. In this instance, we often rely on heuristics and biases to help us quickly navigate patient care. This scenario represents an example of availability bias. The medical student overestimates the probability of the patient having an aortic dissection because the diagnosis of aortic dissection is easy to recall as the medical student just learned about the diagnosis. The medical student judges the likelihood of the event by how easily they could recall the event rather than by carefully assessing the data; this represents availability bias. Omission bias, hindsight bias, and search-satisfying error are all examples of cognitive biases; however, they do not apply to this example. Omission bias is reluctance or avoidance of taking action out of fear of being held responsible for the action. The medical student is not fearful of taking action in this scenario. Hindsight bias is when a practitioner believes he or she accurately predicted the outcome of an event when the correct outcome is known; this limits the practitioner's ability to learn from the past. There is no indication that the medical student in this example is basing the diagnosis on a known outcome. A search-satisfying error is discontinuing a search for an answer when coming across a finding; this did not occur in this case.

Q 6.2: a. Anchoring bias

This example represents anchoring bias where the practitioner makes a decision based on an initial impression and fails to change despite further information. In this example, the pediatrician anchored on a diagnosis of a speech and language disorder and did not consider hearing loss as a possible diagnosis despite minimal progression in appropriate speech-language therapy. Commission bias, regret bias, and availability bias are examples of cognitive biases but do not accurately describe the scenario. Commission bias occurs when the practitioner has a tendency toward action rather than inaction. This is not evident in the current scenario. Regret bias is overestimating the probability of a diagnosis with severe possible consequences because of anticipated regret if the diagnosis was missed. The scenario does not describe regret. In availability bias, the probability of something is overestimated because it is easy to recall. There is no evidence that the physician was recalling a recent case of a speech-language disorder when providing care to the child.

Q 6.3: b. Confirmation bias

This example represents confirmation bias. Confirmation bias is selective data gathering and interpretation of evidence that confirms a diagnosis. In the example, the physician anchored on the diagnosis of pancreatitis. The physician did not take into account the patient's shortness of breath and only ordered a lipase to confirm the diagnostic impression of pancreatitis, thus missing the actual diagnosis of a heart attack. While commission bias, aggregate bias, and regret bias are all examples of cognitive biases they do not accurately describe the scenario. Commission bias occurs when the practitioner has a tendency toward action rather than inaction. In this instance the practitioner does not demonstrate a tendency toward action, such as ordering additional tests or invasive diagnostic procedures.

Aggregate bias is believing a scenario is unusual or atypical, leading a practitioner to ignore guidelines. In this example, the physician believed this was a typical case of pancreatitis and anchored on the diagnosis of acute pancreatitis while ignoring the patient's shortness of breath. Regret bias is overestimating the probability of a diagnosis with severe possible consequences because of anticipated regret if the diagnosis was missed. The scenario does not describe regret, and the physician did not overestimate the probability of a very severe diagnosis as a severe diagnosis (heart attack) was missed.

Q 6.4: d. Search-satisfying error

This example represents a search-satisfying error. In this error, the practitioner discontinues a search for an answer when coming across a finding. The radiologist appropriately diagnosed the lobar pneumonia on the chest X-ray and then inappropriately concluded the search for additional findings. The patient also had an enlarging lung nodule which was missed. While hindsight bias, omission bias, and sunk-cost effect/bias are all examples of cognitive biases they are not represented in this scenario. Hindsight bias is when a practitioner believes he or she accurately predicted the outcome of an event when the correct outcome is known; this limits the practitioner's ability to learn from the past. Omission bias is reluctance or avoidance of taking action out of fear of being held responsible for the action. The radiologist did not take any action in this case and thus this bias is not applicable. Sunk-cost effect/bias occurs when so much has been invested in a decision that a practitioner persists with it. There is no evidence of prior investment in this decision on the part of the radiologist.

Case 7 answers

Q 7.1: d. Payment for services are denied that are a result of a diagnostic error

The eight goals identified in the 2015 Institute of Medicine report, "Improving Diagnosis in Healthcare," for reducing common error are:

1. Facilitate more effective teamwork in the diagnostic process among health care professionals, patients, and their families.
2. Enhance health care professional education and training in the diagnostic process.
3. Ensure the health information technologies (IT) support patients and health care professionals in the diagnostic process.
4. Establish a work system and culture that supports the diagnostic process and improvements in diagnostic performance.
5. Develop a reporting environment and medical liability system that facilitates improved diagnosis through learning from diagnostic errors and near misses.
6. Design a payment and care delivery environment that supports the diagnostic process.
7. Provide dedicated funding for research on the diagnostic process and diagnostic errors.
8. Implementation of these core goals would not only reduce diagnostic errors but also many other medical errors and go a long way toward improving patient safety.

Payment for services that are denied as a result of a diagnostic error would not support goal number 6 in designing a payment and care delivery environment that supports the diagnostic process. Teamwork, partnering with patients and their families, and the utilization of IT are all goals that are aimed at reducing common errors associated with diagnostic errors.

Q 7.2: d. A surgeon uses an incorrectly sterilized instrument during a surgery. The patient subsequently develops a severe bacterial infection and dies

A negligent adverse event is a preventable adverse event where the practitioner did not provide the standard of care of an average practitioner. Malpractice is a negligent adverse event; however, not all negligent adverse events are malpractice. For an event to be considered malpractice, it must be a negligible adverse event where there was a doctor–patient relationship, the negligence contributed to the injury, and the injury led to specific damages. In the example, a surgeon who used an incorrectly sterilized instrument during a surgery is a negligent adverse event as this was a preventable error where the standard of care was violated. Furthermore, the surgeon and patient have a relationship, the surgeon's negligence (using an improperly sterilized instrument) led to the injury (severe bacterial infection), and the injury led to damages (the patient's death). For answer choice a, the patient received the standard of care and suffered an adverse event. For answer choice b, the patient received the standard of care and suffered an adverse event. Having a heart attack during general anesthesia is a known complication, and there is no indication that the standard of care was violated. For answer choice c, the patient received the standard of care. There was no negligence in the case and thus no malpractice.

Case 8 answers

Q 8.1: a. Have everyone introduce themselves and their role in patient care and then provide the purpose and ground rules for the meeting

When an event analysis needs to be conducted, emotions can run high and affect the entire team, unit, and organization. The facilitator of the event analysis must skillfully manage the meeting with compassion and empathy. Creating psychologic safety is essential during this time to allow for individuals to willingly contribute to the conversation without fear of retaliation or humiliation. To create a safe environment, the facilitator should communicate the purpose and goals of the meeting, strengths and knowledge of team members, and an action plan to guide future efforts in creating a safe environment. To start the meeting, the facilitator should have participants introduce themselves and their role in patient care. The facilitator should state the purpose of the meeting and the ground rules of the meeting, such as respecting the opinions of others, not assigning blame, referring to roles and not individual names, and being open to learning and improving care. The facilitator should avoid immediately starting with ground rules, process flow maps, or completed action plans. The facilitator should take the time to create a psychologically safe space by gently starting the meeting with introductions, discussing participants' value in the process, and recreating the scenario in a nonjudgmental manner that allows for active dialogue between participants. From this discussion, an action plan can be developed with input from the team to minimize this type of error from happening again.

Q 8.2: a. For each action item, assign a person to be responsible for ensuring that it is completed

During action planning, the facilitator should foster a discussion around actionable items that are likely to reduce the identified vulnerabilities. For example, stronger action items would include applying human factors, principles, or facility structural changes as opposed to weaker action items such as instituting policies, operating procedures, or trainings. In developing an action plan that promotes a Just Culture, the facilitator should assign individual participants action items to be completed. Developing a 30-, 60-, 90-day plan is important, but the report should be directed toward the manager and leadership so identified barriers can be resolved. Asking for a volunteer to share the lessons learned at the next mortality, morbidity, and improvement conference is premature as more time may be needed to conduct rapid cycles of improvement to determine the best course of action going forward. The facilitator should remind individuals to use titles or roles and not individuals' names and mitigate negative statements during the review of the event, but this does not typically occur during the action planning process.

Suggested further readings

1. Barach P, Small SD. Reporting and preventing medical mishaps: lessons from non-medical near miss reporting systems. *BMJ.* 2000;320:759-763.
2. Dana-Farber Cancer Institute. Principles of a fair and Just Culture. <http://www.ihi.org/resources/Pages/Tools/PrinciplesofaFairandJustCulture.aspx>; 2005 Accessed 24.09.18.
3. Institute for Safe Medication Practices. Building patient safety skills: common pitfalls when conducting a root cause analysis. <https://www.ismp.org/resources/building-patient-safety-skills-common-pitfalls-when-conducting-root-cause-analysis>; 2010 Accessed 24.09.18.
4. Meadows S, Baker K, Butler J. The incident decision tree: guidelines for action following patient safety incidents. In Henriksen K, Battles JB, Marks ES, et al., eds. *Advances in Patient Safety: From Research to Implementation* (Volume 4: Programs, Tools, and Products. Rockville, MD: Agency for Healthcare Research and Quality (US); 2005 Feb. Available from: https://www.ncbi.nlm.nih.gov/books/NBK20586/
5. Morello RT, Lowthian JA, Barker AL, McGinnes R, Dunt D, Brand C. Strategies for improving patient safety culture in hospitals: a systematic review. *BMJ Qual Saf.* 2013;22(1):11-18.
6. Partners HealthCare System. Decision tree for unsafe acts culpability. In Reason J, ed. *Managing the Risks of Organizational Accidents.* Hampshire, England: Ashgate

Publishing Limited; 1997. <http://www.ihi.org/resources/Pages/Tools/DecisionTreeforUnsafeActsCulpability.aspx>; Accessed 24.09.18.

7. National Patient Safety Foundation. *RCA2: Improving Root Cause Analyses and Actions to Prevent Harm.* Boston: National Patient Safety Foundation; 2015.

8. van Klei WA, Hoff RG, van Aarnhem EE, et al. Effects of the introduction of the WHO "surgical safety checklist" on in-hospital mortality: a cohort study. *Ann Surg.* 2012;255(1):44-49.

9. U.S. Department of Veterans Affairs. Root cause analysis tools: VA National Center for Patient Safety. <https://www.patientsafety.va.gov/docs/joe/rca_tools_2_15.pdf>; 2015 Accessed 24.09.18.

8

Quality Improvement

Cecelia Theobald, MD, MPH, Heather Ridinger, MD

Cases and questions

Case 1

Olivia is a third-year medical student hoping to match into a general surgery residency program. She is interested in quality improvement and has been working with a mentor to find a project that would allow her to improve the care of surgical patients. She and her faculty mentor have settled on an improvement idea to decrease the rate of postoperative deep venous thrombosis (DVT).

Q 1.1: Which of the following statements represents a quality improvement initiative designed to reduce the rate of postoperative DVT?

a. A multiinstitutional cohort study comparing the rates of DVT in postoperative patients receiving prevention with either compression devices, ambulation, or heparin
b. A prospective randomized controlled trial comparing the rates of DVT among patients receiving a novel preventive medication compared to the standard of care
c. Implementing a voluntary anonymous survey for all postoperative care nursing staff inquiring about barriers to implementing DVT prevention
d. A chart abstraction of compliance with established DVT prevention protocols followed by a tailored nursing education campaign

Case 2

Hung is a nurse manager at the hepatology clinic. Her staff includes a physician assistant who often sees patients with end-stage liver disease that require large-volume paracentesis to avoid shortness of breath and fluid overload. The nursing staff who assist in these office procedures have commented to her that it is a shame that the paracentesis kits they use come only as a complete bundle. Whenever they need any additional supplies, they have to open another complete set, wasting the remainder of the supplies in the bundle when they go unused. Hung has been thinking about ways to improve the quality of care and decrease the cost. She is interested in designing a quality improvement initiative aimed at reducing unnecessary waste associated with paracenteses in her clinic.

Q 2.1: Which of the following National Academy of Medicine (formerly Institute of Medicine) dimensions of quality health care is most applicable to her quality improvement idea?

a. Safe
b. Timely
c. Effective
d. Efficient
e. Equitable
f. Patient centered

Case 3

Mario is a medical student on an emergency medicine rotation. He has noticed that during the workup for patients in the emergency department, they often receive unnecessary testing or repeat testing that was already done by the referring provider's office or by emergency responders prior to arrival. He knows that health care costs in the United States are increasing and there is a focus on curbing health care–related spending by focusing on quality, cost, and value. He can't help but think that the unnecessary testing ordered by emergency medicine physicians is contributing to increased health care costs.

Q 3.1: Which of the following statements best characterizes the relationship between quality, cost, and value in health care?

a. As quality increases, cost of care decreases
b. Quality seeks to optimize high-value care

c. Quality is defined as the cost for value

d. High-quality care is independent of cost

Case 4

Caroline is a patient safety officer for her hospital, and she is concerned with monitoring a variety of patient safety concerns. She routinely monitors the number of falls occurring in the hospital by evaluating the number of events that are recorded in the hospital's event reporting database. She has noticed that inpatient falls on the geriatric ward have increased over the last 6 months, and she is interested in reducing the rates of inpatient falls.

Q 4.1: What type of data source is she using to gather baseline data?

a. Abstracted

b. Administrative

c. Direct observation

d. Registries

e. Surveillance

Case 5

Eli is a cardiology fellow and interested in evaluating 30-day readmission rates for heart failure patients over the past 10 years. He would like to evaluate what clinical and socioeconomic factors influence whether a patient will be readmitted within 30 days of discharge.

Q 5.1: Which of the following data sources would best suit his project?

a. Administrative

b. Chart review

c. Registries

d. Surveillance

e. Survey

Case 6

Amol is a resident in obstetrics and gynecology at a large tertiary care center and is working with a faculty mentor to implement delayed umbilical cord clamping for 30 to 60 seconds after delivery of very-low-birthweight (VLBW) infants, in accordance with the American College of Obstetricians and Gynecologists and the American Academy of Pediatrics 2012 joint recommendations. These recommendations were based on evidence that VLBW newborns showed improved hemoglobin stores and therefore less need for blood transfusions when delayed umbilical cord clamping was initiated. This initiative would require a coordinated, multidisciplinary approach to improving quality.

Q 6.1: Before beginning the quality improvement project, what next step should Amol take to ensure that he chooses appropriate quality measures?

a. Develop inclusion and exclusion criteria and a protocol for the study based on the existing recommendations

b. Talk with hospital leadership to discuss what they want to measure and gain buy-in for the change

c. Review the existing literature for studies indicating what measures are improved with delayed cord clamping

d. Review outcomes data available in the electronic health record (EHR) for preterm infants at his hospital over the last year

Q 6.2: Amol and his mentor discussed the project and together they developed an aim statement, which was to decrease the transfusion rate of preterm infants by 10% after implementation of delayed cord clamping. After their discussion, Amol decided to track three measures: compliance with the delayed cord clamping protocol, transfusion rates in preterm infants, and admissions for hypothermia in infants who received the delayed cord clamping intervention. Measuring protocol compliance is an example of what type of quality measure?

a. Structural measure

b. Process measure

c. Outcome measure

d. Balancing measure

Q 6.3: Measuring transfusion rate is an example of what type of quality measure?

a. Structural measure

b. Process measure

c. Outcome measure

d. Balancing measure

Q 6.4: Amol is aware that delayed cord clamping can result in infant hypothermia, which sometimes requires escalation of care. He decides to measure admissions for hypothermia, which is an example of which type of quality measure?

a. Structural measure

b. Process measure

c. Outcome measure

d. Balancing measure

Case 7

Barbara is a 67-year-old female with severe primary osteoarthritis in both knees. She has come to a primary care clinic to discuss treatment options, including knee replacement surgery. She is understandably anxious about undergoing such a large surgery and wants to understand all the risks involved. She looks to her physician and asks, "How can I know that I am getting the hospital with the best outcomes?"

Q 7.1: Which of the following can help Barbara make an informed choice about where to get her knee replaced?

a. Centers for Medicare and Medicaid Services (CMS) website

b. Healthcare Bluebook website

c. Heathgrades online reviews

d. Hospital Consumer Assessment of Healthcare Providers and Systems (HCAHPS) survey

e. Medicare Provider Analysis and Review (MedPAR)

Q 7.2: Barbara had an uncomplicated knee replacement surgery 2 months ago, and she is now returning to your clinic. She is very pleased with not only the result of her surgery but also the way she was treated by the entire interprofessional team of providers at the hospital. She is eager to tell you that she has already completed the HCAHPS patient satisfaction survey. Which of the following reasons best describes the role of patient satisfaction data obtained through the HCAHPS care as a quality measure?

a. Patient satisfaction data are reliable sources for identifying and measuring disparities in health care delivery and quality

b. National benchmarks and objective measures of patient satisfaction allow for accountability and comparison between hospitals

c. Patient-derived quality metrics are not used for promotion and insurance reimbursement purposes and therefore are more objective than other measures

d. Patient satisfaction data should not be used as an independent quality metric because of inherent bias

Q 7.3: Which of the following represents a SMART aim statement?

a. We will increase HIV screening among our uninsured patients to detect infection and offer HIV treatment sooner

b. We will improve the percentage of our uninsured clinic patients who have had at least one lifetime HIV screening test to 100% by offering free screenings at a number of sites around the city

c. We will improve the percentage of our uninsured clinic patients who have had at least one lifetime HIV screening test by 20% by December 31 of this year

d. We will improve the rate of HIV detection in the uninsured population by offering free screenings at a number of sites around the city

Q 7.4: Which of the following is TRUE about the process of using Plan-Do-Study-Act (PDSA) cycles for quality improvement?

a. PDSA cycles often begin as a small pilot intervention or test of change and are repeated with slight modifications to allow iterative change

b. PDSA cycles are generally repeated two to four times without changing the intervention in order to allow more rigorous study of the effects

c. After PDSA cycle(s) are planned, the team should define metrics and craft a SMART aim statement

d. PDSA cycles represent a stand-alone quality improvement technique that is generally not combined with other methodologies

Q 7.5: Which of the following best describes the use of Lean methodology for quality improvement?

a. If the proportion of waste in the process can be kept at a constant (no increase), expansion of the process will result in increased value added

b. Value stream mapping is a specific Lean tool that is determined from the viewpoint of the patient (the health care customer) to increase the overall value for a given process

c. Waste of movement is the most common type of health care waste and quality improvement teams should focus their efforts on identifying this

d. The first step in Lean improvement is to identify all the steps in the desired future state process

Case 8

Marco is a pharmacist working to improve the proportion of patients with diabetic nephropathy who are on an angiotensin-converting enzyme (ACE) inhibitor or angiotensin receptor blocker (ARB). His team has chosen a Six Sigma approach to their project.

Q 8.1: What is the usual order of the five steps of the Six Sigma improvement cycle that Marco's team will apply?

a. Define, measure, analyze, improve, control

b. Define, improve, measure, analyze, control

c. Define, analyze, improve, control, measure

d. Analyze, improve, define, measure, control

Q 8.2: Which of the following tools is likely to help Marco's team understand the root causes that have contributed to the current state?

a. Five Whys

b. Fishbone or Ishikawa diagram

c. SWOT analysis

d. Both a and b

Case 9

Chu is a surgeon who has observed significant variation between hospitals in rates of postsplenectomy vaccine administration. She wishes to minimize this variation and ensure that every patient receives all recommended vaccines.

Q 9.1: Which of these quality improvement methodologies would be the most effective for her to use?

a. IHI Model for Improvement

b. Lean

c. Theory of Constraints

d. Six Sigma

Case 10

Danny is the medical director of a small hospice unit whose team wants to work to improve the process for management of end-of-life pain. They are in agreement about the subject but need some help to define an aim and appropriate metrics to measure success.

Q 10.1: Which of these quality improvement methodologies would be the most effective for this team to begin their work?

a. IHI Model for Improvement

b. Lean

c. Theory of Constraints

d. Six Sigma

Case 11

Kaitlyn is a pathologist who learns that their outpatient lab has to repeat up to 10% of labs due to misprocessing by the lab staff, at a significant annual cost. Patients have also complained about the slow rate of lab results. Kaitlyn wants to simplify the redundant current process in an effort to eliminate waste and improve the value the lab offers to the patient.

Q 11.1: Which of these quality improvement methodologies would be the most effective for her team to use in these efforts?

a. IHI Model for Improvement

b. Lean

c. Theory of Constraints

d. Six Sigma

Case 12

Sebastian is an informatics fellow who has developed a clinical decision support tool to help providers in his hospital avoid dangerous drug–drug interactions by warning providers when they try to order two medications that may interact with each other. His tool opens a popup box that prevents providers from ordering the second medication and advises them to discontinue one of the medications before proceeding. He believes this project has great potential impact because the database they are using to determine when drug–drug interactions occur has over 10,000 potential interactions which will trigger an alert.

Q 12.1: Which of the following accurately describes the potential effect of this clinical decision support tool?

a. Providers will likely embrace these alerts as an opportunity to improve patient care

b. The tool will result in more timely administration of medications to patients

c. Due to the large number of warnings that will be generated, there is a high risk of alert fatigue that may lead to work-arounds and cause distraction

d. A more general alert to providers to "review all medications for drug–drug interactions" is more likely to result in improved patient safety

Case 13

Luis is a primary care physician tasked with assessing whether his clinic should adopt a nurse-initiated protocol for ordering mammograms for breast cancer screening. He is concerned that the proposed protocol may increase inappropriate screening for women who do not have indications for screening or do not desire to be screened.

Q 13.1: Which of the following is true with regard to the use of this proposed protocol?

a. All screening orders for mammograms should be standardized and follow this protocol strictly, without exception, to achieve the highest quality care

b. A protocol like this can be useful to minimize unnecessary variations in care as long as physicians are free to personalize care when situations warrant

c. The physician should be allowed to independently decide what screening tests the patient needs, based on his or her training and without the interference of protocols such as these, which are ineffective

d. If used, the screening protocol should be maintained separately from the EHR so as not to confuse care

Case 14

Donna is an anesthesia resident who observed an incident where her patient's intravenous medication was inadvertently attached to the epidural catheter and incorrectly administered via the wrong route. She wants to propose a quality solution that would minimize or eliminate the risk of this critical error occurring again.

Q 14.1: Which of the following is mostly likely to eliminate this error for future patients?

a. Designing the epidural catheter so that it is physically incompatible with the intravenous catheter, preventing the two from being physically joined together

b. Posting reminders on all patient medication bags for staff to double check the intended route of administration prior to beginning infusions

c. Designing a comprehensive education program to education staff about the risks of inadvertent administration of medications via the incorrect route

d. Instituting a checklist for all health care workers to use when they hook up a new medication to provide a reminder to ensure the correct route

Case 15

Bob is the medical director of an outpatient surgery center. He wants to provide useful practice feedback to his colleague, Dr. Greene, on his rates of postoperative surgical site infections, which are slightly above those of his peers.

Q 15.1: Which of the following strategies is most likely to result in effective performance feedback?

a. Asking the clinic nurse administrator to schedule a meeting with Dr. Greene and disclose that his rates are higher than his peers

b. Provide one summary rate for the last 3 years of outcomes

c. Provide his recent value, the target value for the clinic, and suggest action steps

d. Deliver data via email only, to prevent him from missing critical clinical time

Case 16

Amelia is a nurse practitioner working in a community acquired immunodeficiency syndrome (AIDS) clinic in an urban area. She has noticed that many of the clinic's patients miss appointments, which often leads to lapses in their antiviral prescriptions and worse clinical outcomes. She has tried a number of changes to try to improve her own no-show rate, including reaching out to patients ahead of time with text message and phone call reminders. The reminder initiative has been successful at decreasing her no-show rate from 39% to 12% over the past 12 weeks. She is eager to keep this initiative going but finds that the phone calls take a lot of her time. She has reached out to other providers in the clinic about adopting this change clinic-wide but has been met with doubt and lack of motivation to make this change.

Q 16.1: Which of the following is the best next step to assist Amelia in leading this change?

a. Speaking with other providers and clinic staff one-on-one to improve motivation

b. Organizing a clinic staff meeting to share data showing evidence of improvement

c. Working with clinic management to automate the reminder phone calls

d. Offering to personally make the clinic phone calls for other providers' patients

Case 17

Carmen has just completed a project where she led her pediatrics clinic team to improve human papillomavirus (HPV) vaccination rates among adolescents and wants to prepare this work for publication.

Q 17.1: Which of the following is TRUE regarding the publication of her manuscript?

a. No standardized guidelines exist for the reporting of quality improvement scholarship

b. Quality improvement projects can be written up using the same model and guidelines as are used for randomized controlled trials

c. If her intervention changed over the course of the study period, it will be difficult to report this in a rigorous scholarly manner

d. It is important to include information on the context in which the intervention was employed so that readers can assess whether it will apply to their clinical environment

Answers

Case 1 answers

Q 1.1: d. A chart abstraction of compliance with established DVT prevention protocols followed by a tailored nursing education campaign

Quality improvement (QI) is the "systematic and continuous actions that lead to measurable improvement in health care services and the health status of targeted patient groups." QI is often confused with research. Although research and QI share many of the same methods, the purpose of QI differs from that of research. The purpose of QI is to improve the care of the patients, often using evidence-based medicine as a guide. Research, on the other hand, is designed to create new knowledge or discover something that is not already known. In this example, the only option that is NOT a research project is option d. Option a is a multiinstitutional study and is designed to answer the question of which intervention is best. Option b is also research because it is testing a new medicine against the standard of care. Option c is also a study because it requires voluntary consent for participation.

Case 2 answers

Q 2.1: d. Efficient

Efficiency is about reducing unnecessary waste in the systems of care and streamlining care.

Case 3 answers

Q 3.1: b. Quality seeks to optimize high-value care

Quality and value are linked but they are not the same. The definition of value is quality of care divided by the total cost of care. Quality takes into account a number of dimensions, including safety, timeliness, effectiveness, efficiency, equity, and patient centeredness. While reducing waste and streamlining the processes of care all contribute to quality, cost reduction is not always a consideration. Instead, optimizing value (which takes into account cost) is of prime importance in quality improvement work.

Case 4 answers

Q 4.1: e. Surveillance

She is surveilling the hospital's institutional database looking at a specific population of patients as a whole. Abstracted data are derived from patient charts, often based on billing codes and claims. Administrative data refer to publicly reported data from insurance claims or charts. Registries refer to organizations that collect and maintain large, usually nationwide databanks of information about specific populations (e.g., heart failure, cancer, stroke). Direct observation refers to personally observing behaviors or protocols in action (e.g., handwashing compliance).

Case 5 answers

Q 5.1: c. Registries

Quality data can be a rich source of information, not only for quality improvement projects but also for research purposes. Registry data are collected and maintained by a central clearinghouse and analyzed for trends. Registry data contain a rich source of clinical information, not only claims data, as with administrative data sources such as Medicare Provider Analysis Review (MedPAR). With chart review, it would be very difficult to collect for information about the number of patients he will need. Surveillance or surveys will not answer his research question.

Case 6 answers

Q 6.1: c. Review the existing literature for studies indicating what measures are improved with delayed cord clamping

Before any measurement occurs, ask the question, "How will we know that a change is an improvement?" With this question in mind, there are a number of ways to determine the best quality measures to evaluate. Those looking to implement quality improvement will want to choose one or more measures before even evaluating the baseline data. In this way, a quality improvement team can determine the state of things *before* embarking on any change. In this case, Amol will need to review the literature to determine what impact delayed cord clamping is expected to have on VLBW infants before he can determine what measures to evaluate. While hospital leadership buy-in is important to the success of the intervention, it is best to first consider recommendations and expected outcomes based on existing evidence. Existing evidence-based recommendations are always an easy place to begin any quality improvement project.

Q 6.2: b. Process measure

Process measures measure processes carried out by health care professionals in delivering the services of interest. Sometimes process measures are used as surrogate measurements in cases where outcomes are difficult or even impossible to measure. Other times process measures are used to ensure the process is implemented in the intended way. Protocol compliance rates in this case will help Amol know whether there are barriers in implementing the recommendations as he envisions and could inform additional iterations of the change.

Q 6.3: c. Outcome measure

Transfusion rate is the outcome of interest based on Amol's aims statement, so this is the outcome measure in this scenario. Outcome measures are defined as the health outcome of interest. In this case, the outcome is avoiding an intervention (transfusion), so this is the health outcome in this population of VLBW infants.

Q 6.4: d. Balancing measure

Balancing measures are used to ensure the change does not result in any unintended consequences or harm. In this case, Amol is trying to determine if there are unintended harms to infants after initiation of the delayed cord clamping protocol. Structural measures are readily available and related to the structure of the facility or clinical unit being evaluated. Examples in this case may include nurse-to-patient ratios, number of beds in the unit, and number and variety of providers working in the unit, among others.

Case 7 answers

Q 7.1: a. Centers for Medicare and Medicaid Services (CMS) website

Centers for Medicare and Medicaid Services (CMS) website (https://www.cms.gov/) derives publicly reported data into the Hospital Compare website that lists surgical complication rates compared to national averages. A number of other government agencies and private organizations may be helpful to gather publically reported outcomes data (complication rates, number of cases, etc.). The Healthcare Bluebook (https://www.healthcarebluebook.com/) is a publically available resource for patients that helps families make cost-conscious care decisions, but contains no clinical outcomes data. Other online physician reviews such as those found on Healthgrades (https://www.healthgrades.com/) are often from a limited sample of patients and may contain biased or incomplete information and also lack any outcomes data for physicians or hospitals. The HCAHPS is the most widely used patient experience survey but is limited to patient satisfaction data. MedPAR is an administrative databank for claims submitted on Medicare beneficiaries and often contains out-of-date information and is used for population-level research and quality improvement initiatives rather than individual clinical care decisions.
https://www.medicare.gov/hospitalcompare/search.html

Q 7.2: b. National benchmarks and objective measures of patient satisfaction allow for accountability and comparison between hospitals

One of the advantages of including patient experience and satisfaction data as a quality measure is the focus on the patient as a critical stakeholder in improving quality and safety. The HCAHPS is a nationwide, independently administered survey that allows hospitals to be compared on established benchmarks with the purpose of holding hospitals accountable for patient satisfaction measures. Patient satisfaction data are not meant to measure disparities in health care but are often used for physician reimbursement and are routinely used as an independent outcome measure.

Q 7.3: c. We will improve the percentage of our uninsured clinic patients who have had at least one lifetime HIV screening test by 20% by December 31 of this year

A high-quality aim statement for a quality improvement project is often described by the SMART acronym: specific, measurable, attainable, relevant, and time bound. This helps to clearly define a project and ensure that success can be consistently measured. Option c includes all these elements. Option a is closer to a more general goal statement and is missing the specific, measurable, and time-bound components. Option b is specific and measurable but may not be attainable. It is often not practical to reach 100% compliance, nor may it be possible to offer free screenings and does not include a time boundary. Option d contains the planned intervention, which is not a requirement, but is not specific and measurable.

Q 7.4: a. PDSA cycles often begin as a small pilot intervention or test of change and are repeated with slight modifications to allow iterative change

Plan-Do-Study-Act cycles are a key part of the quality improvement process. PDSA cycles are designed to allow for rapid, iterative change so that the intervention can be quickly adapted to address barriers and challenges in real time as they are uncovered. It is not critical that PDSA cycles be repeated without interval change; in fact, adaptation is one of the advantages of this process. The required number of PDSA cycles will vary and must be tailored to the needs of the project. Specific metrics and an aim statement should be defined before beginning PDSA cycles. PDSA cycles are a general structure for tests of change and can be used in concert with other quality improvement methodologies (Lean, Six Sigma, etc.).

Q 7.5: b. Value stream mapping is a specific Lean tool that is determined from the viewpoint of the patient (the health care customer) to increase the overall value for a given process

Lean methodology in quality improvement focuses on the elimination of waste in an effort to maximize efficiency and increase value to the health care consumer (patient). Value stream mapping is one specific Lean tool, which includes time and quality estimates for each step, in an effort to better calculate value from the perspective of the customer (in health care, usually the patient). If a process contains any significant amount of waste and the scale of the process is increased without reducing the amount of waste, the overall result will be a magnification of waste. Waste of overproduction, not waste of movement, is generally the most common type of health care waste. The first step in Lean improvement is *process mapping,* or to thoroughly map out the current state as it is without desired changes, to gain a common understanding among the team members (Fig. 8.1).

Case 8 answers

Q 8.1: a. Define, measure, analyze, improve, control
Q 8.2: d. Both a and b

In general, Six Sigma methodology follows a five-step process: define, measure, analyze, improve, control (or DMAIC). Once the team has defined the scope, purpose, and team of the project, they move into the measure phase, where they seek to understand the current state of the process as well as plan for metrics and data collection. Both the fishbone (or Ishikawa) diagram and the Five Whys tool can be used in the measure and analyze phases to better understand the root causes that lead to the problem or current state. SWOT (strengths-weaknesses-opportunities-threats) analysis is another tool that can be used in the measure phase but does not elucidate as much information about root causes (Fig. 8.2).

Specific Quality Improvement Approaches

Methodology	Plan, Do, Study, Act (PDSA)	Lean	Six Sigma
Focus	Structured planning and testing of solutions	Eliminate waste across service lines to improve quality, workflow, and value	Statistical-based problem solving and improvement
Primary Target	Piloting improvements	Workflow	Large problems and variation
Approach	Plan Do Study Act	Value Value Stream Flow Pull Perfection	Define Measure Analyze Improve Control
Primary Result	Improvements through small tests of change	Reduced flow times	Uniform process output

Fig. 8.1 Specific quality improvement approaches. (Source: Kautz JM, Armistead NS, Starr SR. Quality improvement. In Skochelak SE, et al. *Health Systems Science.* Philadelphia: Elsevier Health Sciences; 2016:68–80.)

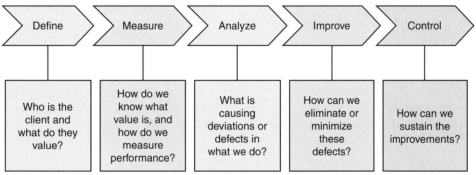

Fig. 8.2 Six Sigma methodology. (Source: Lee CS, Wadhwa V, Kruskal JB, Larson DB. Conducting a successful practice quality improvement project for American Board of Radiology Certification. *Radiograph.* 2015.)

Cases 9, 10, and 11 answers

Q 9.1: d. Six Sigma
Q 10.1: a. IHI Model for Improvement
Q 11.1: b. Lean
Generally speaking, the IHI Model for Improvement is most useful to focus on a structured plan and test iterative solutions via small tests of change. Lean is useful for identifying and eliminating health care waste in an effort to improve value. The Theory of Constraints is a method for identifying critical limiting factor(s) that prevent a goal from being achieved. Six Sigma is a method designed to focus on the reduction of variation and the elimination of undesirable outcomes. Six Sigma would be the most useful to minimize variation in postsplenectomy vaccines and avoid missed vaccines.

Case 12 answers

Q 12.1: c. Due to the large number of warnings that will be generated, there is a high risk of alert fatigue that may lead to work-arounds and cause distraction
Clinical decision support (CDS) tools can provide just-in-time information to providers to increase the quality and safety of care. However, custodians of CDS tools must remain vigilant to ensure alerts are timely, specific, actionable, and significant, or providers will grow weary of the volume of alerts. In some cases, excessive alerts can actually lead to delays in care and administration of medications, such as in this case. Alert fatigue from a large number of clinically insignificant alerts can lead to providers ignoring potentially serious alerts and employing workarounds. Highly specific, clinically relevant alerts are the most likely to result in improved patient safety.

Case 13 answers

Q 13.1: b. A protocol like this can be useful to minimize unnecessary variations in care as long as physicians are free to personalize care when situations warrant
Unnecessary variation in health care practices is common. Protocol-based care can improve unacceptable variation in patient care. It is important that when utilized, protocols allow providers to opt out of protocol-recommended care if patient-specific factors or system factors dictate that care recommended by the protocol is inappropriate. Furthermore, protocolized care is most effective when it is embedded into the EHR.

Case 14 answers

Q 14.1: a. Designing the epidural catheter so that it is physically incompatible with the intravenous catheter, preventing the two from being physically joined together

Although there are occasions where reminders, education, and checklists can be part of successful quality and safety campaigns, these methods allow busy or distracted staff to occasionally make errors. When possible, equipment redesign (such as changing the epidural catheter so it is not physically compatible with the wrong line) is an example of a forcing function that prevents individuals from making mistakes and relies less on memory/intention.

Case 15 answers

Q 15.1: c. Provide his recent value, the target value for the clinic, and suggest action steps

Audit and performance feedback can be a powerful change tool for quality improvement but must be delivered in an actionable and useful manner. Effective feedback tends to be provided repeatedly with trends, in both verbal and written forms, by a colleague or direct supervisor, and paired with actionable steps as well as specific targets.

Case 16 answers

Q 16.1: c. Working with clinic management to automate the reminder phone calls

Change management is often a difficult part of the change process, and successful interventions require a coordinated and thoughtful approach to change management within the organization. Some of the change concepts that are important to remember are connecting to motivation, making the right thing easy to do, offering reward and recognition in a meaningful way, and fostering an environment of engagement for all. Working with the clinic manager to make the phone calls and texts the easy thing to do would likely go the furthest toward improving motivation and buy-in among the clinic staff. Amelia has already reached out to discuss her initiative with other providers and was met with doubt, so speaking one-on-one again without any meaningful improvement in the process will be a less effective approach.

Case 17 answers

Q 17.1: d. It is important to include information on the context in which the intervention was employed so that readers can assess whether it will apply to their clinical environment

The process of telling the story of improvement work often requires a different approach and organization than is used in research. The SQUIRE 2.0 guidelines provide a comprehensive and widely accepted checklist for high-quality reporting of improvement initiatives. One of the key features of SQUIRE is a focus on providing information about the context of an intervention, so that readers can more easily determine what changes may need to be applied prior to application in their own environment. Furthermore, quality improvement reporting guidelines provide the flexibility for an intervention to evolve as it is deployed.

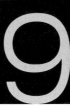

Teamwork and Collaboration

Kelly Caverzagie, MD, Devin Nickol, MD

Cases and questions

Case 1

A 73-year-old woman is admitted to the hospital from home for a scheduled right hip replacement. Her past medical history is significant for hypertension, osteoarthritis, type 2 diabetes, and mild dementia.

Q 1.1: Before surgery, the patient expresses a preference for postoperative discharge to home, rather than to a nursing or rehabilitation facility. Which member of the care team is most qualified to assess the patient's ability to independently perform her activities of daily living at home once she is stabilized postoperatively?
a. Physician
b. Nurse
c. Pharmacist
d. Physical therapist
e. Social worker

Q 1.2: During a previous hospitalization, the patient developed delirium, including agitation and wandering behaviors. The patient and her family inquire about potential measures to decrease her risk of delirium following her hip replacement. Which of the following interventions would be most appropriate to reduce her risk of postoperative delirium?
a. Hydration
b. A delirium prevention team
c. Low-dose haloperidol
d. Low-dose lorazepam
e. Structured patient handoffs

Q 1.3: During her hospitalization, the patient is cared for in an interprofessional geriatric evaluation and management unit (GEMU). Which of the following outcomes is most likely to be improved by this approach?
a. Mortality rate
b. Length of stay
c. Functional decline
d. Readmission rate

Case 2

A large tertiary care hospital has decided to restructure its inpatient ward services. All primary care rounds will be conducted by interdisciplinary teams, which will include a physician, pharmacist, social worker, and nurse coordinator.

Q 2.1: After 1 year of implementation, which of the following patient care metrics is most likely to show improvement?
a. Total cost of stay
b. Inpatient mortality
c. Successful discharge to home
d. Catheter-associated urinary tract infection (UTI)
e. Rate of adverse drug interactions

Q 2.2: Which of the following characteristics will best predict the overall performance of the hospital's newly created interprofessional teams?
a. The average social sensitivity of team members
b. The average intelligence of team members
c. The level of motivation of team members
d. Self-reported satisfaction levels of team members

Case 3

A community hospital provides inpatient surgical care using interprofessional teams that include a physician, a nurse, an occupational therapist, a social worker, and a pharmacist. Each morning, team members meet to review patient progress and assign care tasks for the day. During today's meeting, the team's nurse reports that, in addition to his usual nursing duties, he has been spending large amounts of time on other aspects of patient care. He has helped family members identify and contact local nursing homes and rehabilitation facilities to expedite hospital discharges, and, yesterday, he spent 45 minutes teaching a patient who recently had a knee replacement how to use an extendible reaching device.

Q 3.1: Which of the following concepts in team-based care best addresses this common situation?
a. Excessive autonomy
b. Role blurring
c. Ineffective collaboration
d. Failure to adhere to team ethics

Q 3.2: Which of the following factors impacts the scope of practice (i.e., the activities permissible based on an individual's professional license) of this team's members at the micro level?
a. Coverage of services by insurance
b. Legislation from regulatory bodies addressing scope of practice
c. Practice agreements with local institutions
d. Interpersonal interactions within the team

Case 4

The staff of a stroke rehabilitation center wish to improve the quality of the team-based, interprofessional care they provide to patients. Over a 6-month period, the staff participate in a training program consisting of exercises in case-based problem solving and formative feedback and assessment of team function before and after the training sessions. Participants include physicians, nurses, pharmacists, physical and occupational therapists, and social workers.

Q 4.1: When compared to stroke patients receiving usual care, patients cared for by the staff after their training program are more likely to achieve better results in which of the following areas?
a. Length of stay
b. Successful discharge to home
c. Functional improvement
d. Total cost of hospitalization

Case 5

A hospital decides to implement a care pathway for all patients admitted with exacerbations of chronic obstructive pulmonary disease (COPD). Patients will be cared for by an interprofessional team whose members have received special training in cooperatively managing COPD in the inpatient setting. Team members receive feedback about their performance at baseline and work to identify evidence-based key interventions shown to impact outcomes for patients hospitalized with COPD exacerbations.

Q 5.1: Measurement of team performance 1 year later is most likely to show improvement in which of the following areas?
a. Length of stay
b. Inpatient mortality
c. Risk of provider burnout
d. Total cost of hospitalization

Case 6

The medical leadership of a nursing home becomes concerned about the frequency with which sedative and antipsychotic medications are being used to manage behavioral symptoms among elderly residents. They institute a schedule of monthly, pharmacist-led meetings among the staff. Participants include physicians, nurses, and nursing aides. The meetings focus on interprofessional communication skills, geriatric medication issues, and appropriate management of behavioral symptoms, including avoidance of nonrecommended medications.

Q 6.1: One year later, which of the following outcomes is most likely to be seen among residents of the facility?
a. Fewer antipsychotic medications prescribed
b. Fewer total medications prescribed
c. Decreased fall risk
d. Fewer hospitalizations

Case 7

An outpatient primary care practice institutes a team-based care program involving community pharmacists. Under collaborative practice agreements, practice physicians will refer patients to the program, and pharmacists will help manage the care of patients with certain chronic conditions. Using defined treatment goals, the role of the pharmacists will include monitoring lab values, adjusting medications, and providing patient education.

The first program developed by the practice is designed to improve the care of Medicaid patients with diabetes and hemoglobin A1c levels above goal. A local pharmacist tracks patients' glycemic control and adjusts medication doses. The pharmacist also provides the patients with diabetes-specific disease education and counseling as needed, either in person or by phone. Referrals to the program are initiated by the patient's primary care provider.

Q 7.1: Six months after the initiation of the program, which of the following outcomes is most likely?
a. Decreased cost of care
b. Lower hemoglobin A1c values
c. Less prescription drug use
d. Fewer outpatient visits

Q 7.2: The practice develops a second program to improve blood pressure control for hypertensive patients. Physicians refer patients to the program, and community pharmacists meet independently with the enrolled patients. The pharmacists monitor patients' blood pressures, order any necessary laboratory testing, and provide medication recommendations to the referring physician by phone or fax for approval. The pharmacists provide education and counseling to the patients about treatment options, medication costs, and side effects. After 6 months, when compared to patients managed in a traditional, physician-led clinic, which of the following outcomes is most likely to be observed among patients enrolled in the pharmacist-led hypertension clinic?
a. Fewer overall clinic visits
b. Fewer prescribed medications
c. Lower overall cost of care
d. Lower systolic and diastolic blood pressure
e. Fewer hospitalizations

Case 8

A hospital administrator wishes to implement an interprofessional, collaborative care model to reduce overall hospital mortality rates.

Q 8.1: Which of the following conclusions is she most likely to reach after reviewing high-quality, randomized trials addressing this topic?
a. Prerounding huddles will decrease mortality rates
b. Structured communication tools (e.g., SBAR) will decrease mortality rates
c. A facilitated staff retreat on interprofessional care will decrease mortality rates
d. Interprofessional decision support tools in the EHR will decrease mortality rates
e. No published studies have reported decreased mortality rates when comparing an interprofessional care model to usual care

Case 9

University Health System (UHS) is interested in improving the care of patients transferred from the intensive care unit (ICU) to the general medical-surgical floor. Compared to other similar hospitals, UHS has a high rate of transfer back to the ICU for those who have transferred within the preceding 48 hours, which is due to a lack of communication between caregivers in the ICU and the general floor.

Q 9.1: Which of the following standardized communication strategies could be implemented with the goal of reducing error and improving outcomes?
a. Callout
b. Checkback
c. Handoff
d. SBAR (situation-background-assessment-recommendation)
e. CUS (concerned-uncomfortable-safety)

Q 9.2: A medical-surgical nurse contacts the resident physician on call to notify her that a patient who just transferred from the ICU is having low blood pressures that are new since receiving handoff from the ICU nurse. The elderly patient, admitted to the ICU for pneumonia, has otherwise stable vital signs. The nurse notifies the resident that the patient has already received antibiotics and asks if she should start intravenous fluids. This scenario best describes which type of communication strategy?
a. Callout
b. Checkback
c. Handoff
d. SBAR (situation-background-assessment-recommendation)
e. CUS (concerned-uncomfortable-safety)

Q 9.3: Despite starting intravenous fluids and continuing other cares, the patient's condition deteriorates, and he is now having difficulty breathing with a blood pressure of 88/50, pulse of 120 beats per minute, and an oxygen saturation of 84% on 4 liters oxygen per nasal cannula. The patient has just lost consciousness, and the nurse yells to the hallway for assistance and activates a Code Blue. This scenario best describes which type of communication strategy?
a. Callout
b. Checkback

c. Handoff
d. SBAR (situation-background-assessment-recommendation)
e. CUS (concerned-uncomfortable-safety)

Case 10

A 46-year-old male presents to clinic for a refill of his blood pressure (BP) medications and is found to have a BP of 168/94 mmHg. The resident changes the patient's regimen from amlodipine to extended-release carvedilol once/day and discharges the patient from clinic with instructions to follow up in 1 month. A short while later, the clinic social worker, who has been helping the patient obtain health insurance coverage, asks to see the patient. The resident, proud of his efficiency, describes the plan and states that the patient has already left the clinic. Frustrated, the social worker reminds the resident that the patient cannot afford medicines, especially this new prescription which costs 10 times more than the prior regimen.

Q 10.1: Which of the following preencounter team communication strategies could have prevented this suboptimal patient encounter?
a. Huddle
b. Callout
c. Brief
d. Debrief
e. CUS (concerned-uncomfortable-safety)

Case 11

A 61-year-old female presents to the emergency department with complaints of chest heaviness and difficulty breathing. She has a known history of essential hypertension, type 2 diabetes, and gout. After obtaining a brief history, the nurse establishes an IV, draws bloodwork, and obtains an electrocardiogram (ECG) per hospital protocol. She shows the ECG to the attending physician who is concerned about an acute ST-elevation myocardial infarction. The physician quickly gathers the nurse, resident physician, care tech, and triage nurse and assigns each with responsibilities to care for the patient and activate the cardiac catheterization lab for immediate patient transport.

Q 11.1: Which of the following team communication strategies best describes this scenario?
a. Huddle
b. Callout
c. Brief
d. Debrief
e. CUS (concerned-uncomfortable-safety)

Case 12

With the goal of improving the overall performance of her family medicine clinic, the clinic medical director determines that she will pursue clinic accreditation as a patient-centered medical home (PCMH) care delivery model.

Q 12.1: In a patient-centered medical home model of care, multidisciplinary teams work together to improve care by providing comprehensive care management for a population of patients through tracking and coordination of care while enhancing access

to and continuity of care. Which of the following best describes another key function of a PCMH?
a. Electronic health record (EHR) template
b. Performance management and quality improvement
c. Insurance risk adjustment
d. Pursue alternative reimbursement models
e. Clearinghouse for outpatient procedures and tests

Q 12.2: While working to increase access to and coordinate medical care for a defined population, the PCMH model of care can also reduce the costs of care by doing which of the following?
a. Reducing unnecessary emergency department visits
b. Reducing prescription drug utilization
c. Transitioning clinic practices to provide care to patients who have health insurance
d. Limiting reimbursement to ambulatory clinics
e. Limiting bureaucracy associated with managed care

Q 12.3: As part of establishing the PCMH, the clinic director has all employees and clinicians complete formalized team training. In clinics that have established a strong team culture, the development of tight team structures can lead to which of the following?
a. Decreased clinician exhaustion
b. Decreased staff exhaustion
c. Greater clinical revenue
d. Greater team social interaction
e. Decreased patient no-show rate

Case 13

Dr. Thompson is the new chief executive officer (CEO) for University Medicine, the large community-based health system affiliated with a medical school. Through her meetings and observations, it becomes clear that hospital administrators, physicians, and other members of the care delivery team are not working together as a team to achieve better outcomes for patients and populations. She assigns Dr. Richards, the chief patient experience officer, to develop a plan to transform the culture of the health system to think like and function as a team.

Q 13.1: In her work, Dr. Richards reflects upon how to lead this transformation. She recalls that leadership is multifaceted and that good leaders demonstrate differing leadership approaches depending upon the environment. For this situation, Dr. Richards decides to take a supportive approach where she is considerate of those on her team and provides structure through task-oriented direction. Which leadership approach best describes Dr. Richards's approach?
a. Relational
b. Transformational
c. Behavioral
d. Transactional
e. Contingency

Q 13.2: To achieve her goal, Dr. Richards must work to optimize team effectiveness. Evidence from fields outside of medicine reveals that effective team interactions are comprised of cognitive, affective, and behavioral processes. Which of the following best represents a cognitive team process?
a. Team development of a shared mental model of goals and responsibilities

b. Development of team interdependence leading to cohesion
c. Similar perceptions about team efficacy
d. Allocation of resources to perform tasks and adapt to changing goals
e. Development of team-oriented knowledge, skills, and attitudes

Case 14

Patients cared for in the ICU require an extensive team of providers and other personnel to deliver life-supporting therapies with a goal toward recovery.

Q. 14.1 When utilized as members of the ICU care team, evidence suggests that family members can positively affect which of the following?
a. Avoidance of ICU delirium
b. Maintenance of nutrition
c. Recovery of physical function
d. Long-term psychologic outcomes
e. Reduction of disease burden

Case 15

In the ICU, implementation of an evidence-based set of guidelines known as the ABCDEF bundle significantly improves outcomes in patients who are on mechanical ventilation. Despite these positive results, implementation of this bundle is incomplete in many ICUs. Many barriers to implementation exist and focus on issues related to patients, clinicians, protocols, and other contextual factors.

Q 15.1: Which of the following strategies is most likely to require significant care team coordination to overcome a common barrier?
a. Identify screening tools to choose patients who will benefit
b. Develop specific protocols for use by the interprofessional care team
c. Improve team member knowledge of the ABCDEF bundle
d. Synchronize interprofessional staffing and work scheduling
e. Educate patient and family about the interprofessional team

Answers

Case 1 answers

Q 1.1: d. Physical therapist
The physical therapist (PT) is best qualified to take the lead in assessing the patient's physical abilities at the time of discharge, although other professions may take on a portion of this responsibility as well. The other professions mentioned will also have important discharge-related roles to fulfill, but the patient's recent hip replacement means that mobility issues are likely to have the greatest impact on her ability to manage her activities of daily living at home. The PT is best suited to assume the leadership role in evaluating her functional abilities.

Q 1.2: b. A delirium prevention team

The multicomponent, collaborative, nonpharmacologic interventions offered by a delirium prevention team can prevent delirium in older hospitalized patients. These interventions are intended to identify and address delirium risk factors such as sleep deprivation and impairments in mobility, vision, or hearing. In the research project cited, the team consisted of a geriatrician, a nurse, a physical therapist, and representatives of other professions with specialized geriatric training. Many commonly used pharmacologic agents, including antipsychotic medications (haloperidol) and sedatives (lorazepam), have been studied and either increase delirium risk or fail to reduce the risk. Other interventions (e.g., hydration) have been poorly studied and have not been shown to have benefit. Structured patient handoffs are intended to improve the quality of team-based care and prevent medical errors but have not been shown to impact the risk of delirium.

Suggested further reading

1. Inouye SK, Bogardus Jr ST, Charpentier PA, et al. A multicomponent intervention to prevent delirium in hospitalized older patients. *New Engl J Med*. 1999;340(9): 669-676.

Q 1.3: c. Functional decline

A geriatric evaluation and management unit (GEMU) is an inpatient unit designed to provide interprofessional care to elderly patients. Investigators in the study referenced performed a meta-analysis of existing research and found that patients cared for in a GEMU setting demonstrated better functional status at discharge and a lower rate of institutionalization (e.g., nursing home placement) at 1 year. There was no significant impact on mortality, readmission rate, or length of stay. Additional research in this area is needed; however, there is some evidence that specialized units providing effective, team-based care may offer advantages for specific patient populations, including the frail elderly.

Case 2 answers

Q 2.1: a. Total cost of stay

To date, relatively few studies have formally evaluated the effect of interprofessional care teams in the inpatient setting. Evidence of benefit has not been demonstrated for metrics, including mortality; discharge to home; nosocomial infections, including UTI; or medical errors, including adverse drug interactions. Interprofessional care may result in small decreases in length of stay and associated decreases in the total cost of hospitalization.

Suggested further reading

1. Curley C, McEachern JE, Speroff T. A firm trial of interdisciplinary rounds on the inpatient medical wards: an intervention designed using continuous quality improvement. *Med Care*. 1998;36:AS4-12.

Q 2.2: a. The average social sensitivity of team members

Team function is a complex topic and understanding the dynamic factors that affect the performance of groups of individuals is a challenging task for researchers in the fields of psychology and interprofessional care. Perhaps counterintuitively, studies have shown that team performance (collective intelligence) on a variety of tasks is not strongly correlated with the intelligence, satisfaction, or motivation of individual team members. Performance does seem to be correlated with the social sensitivity of team members (i.e., the ability to work with others) and the ability of the team to allow multiple members to speak and contribute.

Suggested further reading

1. Woolley AW, Chabris CF, Pentland A, Hashmi N, Malone TW. Evidence for a collective intelligence factor in the performance of human groups. *Science*. 2010; 330(6004):686-688.

Case 3 answers

Q 3.1: b. Role blurring

Theoretical discussions in the fields of interprofessional education and collaborative practice often stress the importance of eliminating the isolating effect associated with traditional silos of professional identity and moving to a model of shared responsibilities and team-based care. This loss of clearly drawn boundaries between professions can lead to role blurring where a given care activity could potentially fall under the responsibility of team members from more than one profession. A situation can also arise where the same care issue might be addressed by different team members on different occasions. The results of role blurring can be positive or negative, depending on the setting. The flexibility of operating without strictly assigned turf must be weighed against the possibility of team members being overloaded with responsibilities as a consequence. The principles of autonomy, collaboration, and team ethics are all relevant to the question, but the concept of role blurring combines these to best describe the situation in this scenario.

Suggested further reading

1. Brown B, Crawford P, Darongkamas J. Blurred roles and permeable boundaries: the experience of multidisciplinary working in community mental health. *Health Soc Care Community*. 2000;8(6):425-435.

Q 3.2: d. Interpersonal interactions within the team

One way to categorize scope of practice issues affecting an interprofessional team is to classify them as operating at the micro (within the team), meso (within the institution), or macro (regulatory agency) levels. Team interactions occur at the micro level, institutional arrangements such as practice agreements at the meso level, and issues related to regulatory bodies and coverage of services at the macro level. The real-world function of a given team,

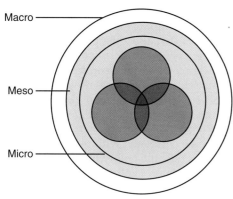

Fig. 9.1 Conceptual model of factors influencing collaborative models of health care. (Bourgeault IL, Mulvale G. Collaborative health care teams in Canada and the USA: confronting the structural embeddedness of medical dominance. *Health Sociol Rev.* 2006;15(5):481–495.)

including the scopes of the roles played by its members, will be determined by interactions between factors operating at all three levels (Fig. 9.1).

Case 4 answers

Q 4.1: c. Functional improvement

The challenges of providing team-based, collaborative care may be justified if it is possible to demonstrate improvement in meaningful outcomes for patients or populations. Research has not yet shown significant improvements in cost, length of stay, or rates of discharge to home when such care is provided in the manner described in the question. Few randomized trials have compared the results of team training to usual care, but the study referenced found evidence of improved functional status among stroke patients cared for by teams that had completed training workshops emphasizing team-based, problem-solving strategies.

Suggested further reading

1. Strasser DC, Falconer JA, Stevens AB, et al. Team training and stroke rehabilitation outcomes: a cluster randomized trial. *Arch Phys Med Rehabil.* 2008;89(1): 10-15.

Case 5 answers

Q 5.1: c. Risk of provider burnout

Provider burnout is an area of increasing concern in clinical medicine. The possibility that enhanced interprofessional teamwork could reduce one or more of the stressors leading to burnout is an attractive one. Care pathways represent a structured approach to the care of patients with complex medical problems and have been used in the management of hospitalized patients with a variety of conditions. Although there is currently no evidence that the intervention described would impact length of stay, mortality, or total costs, research has shown decreased risk of burnout among providers on teams similar to the one described. This may be

due to the perception among team members that they are supported in their role, resulting in an increased ability to cope with the stresses of the work environment.

Suggested further reading

1. Deneckere S, Euwema M, Lodewijckx C, et al. Better interprofessional teamwork, higher level of organized care, and lower risk of burnout in acute health care teams using care pathways: a cluster randomized controlled trial. *Med Care.* 2013;51(1):99-107.

Case 6 answers

Q 6.1: a. Fewer antipsychotic medications prescribed

The presence of patients with complex health care needs, including a large number of comorbidities and a high potential for adverse drug events, makes nursing homes a logical site for collaborative team-based care. Guidelines recommending avoidance of several classes of high-risk drugs in elderly nursing home patients are frequently not followed. The referenced study found that monthly, pharmacist-led staff meetings resulted in a decrease in the number of antipsychotic medications prescribed to manage behavioral symptoms, a change congruent with established guidelines. There was no decrease in the total number of medications prescribed, and no statistically significant change in the rate of falls or hospitalizations.

Suggested further reading

1. Schmidt I, Claesson CB, Westerholm B, Nilsson LG, Svarstad BL. The impact of regular multidisciplinary team interventions on psychotropic prescribing in Swedish nursing homes. *J Am Geriatr Soc.* 1998;46(1):77-82.

Case 7 answers

Q 7.1: b. Lower hemoglobin A1c values

Collaborative practice models based on physician referral of selected patients to pharmacist-led programs have been shown to have positive impacts on multiple disease-specific outcome measures. One such type of program focuses on improvement of glycemic control in diabetic patients through monitoring, counseling, and medication adjustment performed by pharmacists. Although no significant positive effects have been found in the outcomes of cost, decreased number of prescription medications, or number of per capita visits needed, research has shown improvement in glycemic control as measured by the hemoglobin A1c.

Suggested further reading

1. Biltaji E, Yoo M, Jennings BT, Leiser JP, McAdam-Marx C. Outcomes associated with pharmacist-led diabetes collaborative drug therapy management in a Medicaid population. *J Pharm Health Serv Res.* 2017;8(1): 59-62.

Q 7.2: d. Lower systolic and diastolic blood pressure

Similar to the prior scenario, pharmacist-led management of medical treatment of hypertension has been shown to result in lower systolic and diastolic blood pressure among participating patients. The number of clinic visits, prescribed medications, cost of care, and number of hospitalizations did not decrease.

Suggested further readings

1. Carter BL, Rogers M, Daly J, Zheng S, James PA. The Potency of Team-Based Care Interventions for Hypertension: A Meta-analysis. *Arch Intern Med.* 2009; 169(19):1748-1755.
2. Okamoto, MP, Nakahiro, RK. Pharmacoeconomic evaluation of a pharmacist-managed hypertension clinic. *Pharmacotherapy.* 2001;21:1337-1344.

Case 8 answers

Q 8.1: e. No published studies have reported decreased mortality rates when comparing an interprofessional care model to usual care

Interprofessional collaboration (IPC) is a component of many modern practice models, including the patient-centered medical home (PCMH) and accountable care organizations (ACOs). Interprofessional education is now mandated by the accrediting bodies of all major health professions training programs (e.g., Liaison Committee on Medical Education [LCME] for US medical schools). There is increasing interest in the promise of individual and societal benefits that may arise from better teamwork and collaboration among health care providers, including advancement of the Triple Aim (improved experience of care, improved population health, and decreased costs). Periodic reviews of the literature have shown a gradually increasing evidence base in the field of interprofessional practice; however, the number of high-quality trials comparing interprofessional collaborative care to usual care remains low. Although existing studies have been able to show limited benefits of IPC in some specific populations and settings, none have demonstrated a clear mortality benefit using any of the modalities listed in the question. Given the growing investment in IPC from students, providers, patients, and society, there is a clear need for funding for additional research in this area.

Suggested further reading

1. Reeves S, Pelone F, Harrison R, Goldman J, Zwarenstein M. Interprofessional collaboration to improve professional practice and healthcare outcomes. *Cochrane Database Syst Rev.* 2017;6(06):CD000072.

Case 9 answers

Q 9.1: c. Handoff
Q 9.2: d. SBAR (situation-background-assessment-recommendation)
Q 9.3: a. Callout

Information sharing (i.e., communication) between individuals is at the heart of effective team performance. The use of closed-loop communication (where the listener acknowledges receipt of the information and clarifies understanding with the sender) and incorporation of structured communication protocols foster team awareness and clarity. TeamSTEPPS, a widely available teamwork-training course used by many health systems and clinics, introduces several effective individual communication strategies:

- Callout: a technique that informs all team members of an emergent situation (i.e., "I need help in here!"), as in Question 9.3
- Checkback: a technique that uses closed-loop communication between two individuals to ensure the receiver fully understands what the sender intended
- Handoff: the formal transfer of information and authority during a transition of care. Handoffs are more effective if using a standardized format or template throughout an organization. Handoffs are the most influential communication strategy to improve safety, reduce error, and improve patient outcomes, as in Question 9.1
- SBAR (situation-background-assessment-recommendation): a technique for communicating between two individuals to relay critical information that requires action or attention, as in Question 9.2

Cases 10 and 11 answers

Q 10.1: c. Brief
Q 11.1: a. Huddle

Leadership is critical to the success of any team. Historically, physicians have served as the de facto leader in any professional health care setting. However, there are times when the physician may not be the best person to serve in this role, and increasingly health care is shifting to collective team-based care. TeamSTEPPS, a widely available teamwork-training course used by many health systems and clinics, also introduces several effective team-based communication strategies:

- Brief: short gathering of team members prior to the start of a session (e.g., session in a primary care clinic, surgical procedure in operating room) with the goal of sharing the plan, assigning responsibilities, and anticipating outcomes and likely contingencies, as in Question 10.1
- Huddle: an ad hoc meeting to reestablish situational awareness, reinforce plans, and assess the need to adjust the plan, as in Question 11.1
- Debrief: informal information exchange after an event or session to reflect upon lessons learned and reinforce positive behaviors

Suggested further reading

1. TeamSTEPPS 2.0. *Team Strategies & Tools to Enhance Performance & Patient Safety. Curriculum Materials. Essentials Instructional Module and Course Slides.* Agency for Healthcare Research and Quality; 2012. Available at: https://www.ahrq.gov/teamstepps/instructor/essentials/index.html. Updated March 2014. Accessed May 9, 2018.

Case 12 answers

Q 12.1: b. Performance management and quality improvement
Q 12.2: a. Reducing unnecessary emergency department visits

The patient-centered medical home (PCMH) is an evolving care delivery model designed to provide enhanced primary care services that are of value to patients, families, and the care teams who work with both. One key aspect of the PCMH is the incorporation of team-based care principles in which team members are able to work and function at the top of their skill set. The PCMH model provides many benefits to patients, including enhanced access to care, greater community relationships, reduction in health care costs, and/or unnecessary utilization of emergency department visits, inpatient hospitalizations, and hospital readmissions.

The National Committee for Quality Assurance (NCQA) has established standards required of a clinic or practice that seeks to be designated as a PCMH:

1. Practice organized using team-based care principles
2. Understanding and subsequently managing populations of patients
3. Access and continuity of care that is patient centered
4. Assistance and support to help patients manage their care
5. Coordination of care provided by multiple providers and during transitions between settings
6. Performance measurement and quality improvement (Question 12.1)

Suggested further readings

1. Nielsen M, Buelt L, Patel K, Nichols LM. The Patient-Centered Medical Home's Impact on Cost and Quality, Review of Evidence, 2014-2015. 2016. Available at: https://www.pcpcc.org/resource/patient-centered-medical-homes-impact-cost-and-quality-2014-2015. Accessed May 23, 2018.
2. National Committee on Quality Assurance Academy. Introduction to PCMH 2017. Available at: https://www.ncqa.org/Portals/0/Programs/Recognition/Intro_to_PCMH_2017.pdf?ver=2017-11-01-220650-193. Accessed May 23, 2018.

Q 12.3: a. Decreased clinician exhaustion

A cross-sectional survey of clinicians and staff members of 16 primary care clinics revealed that working in a tight team structure and having perceptions of a greater team culture are associated with less clinician exhaustion. While greater team culture was associated with less exhaustion among staff, team structure failed to predict exhaustion among staff.

Suggested further reading

1. Willard-Grace R. Hessler D. Rogers E. Dubé K. Bodenheimer T. Grumbach K. Team structure and culture are associated with lower burnout in primary care. *J Am Board Fam Med.* 2014;27:229-238.

Case 13 answers

Q 13.1: c. Behavioral

Team leadership is multifaceted and variable depending on the situational context and the leaders' individual experience and skills. Leaders' approach to working with their team may vary depending upon the nature of the task and goals for the team, as well as the composition for the team. Physicians should demonstrate varying approaches to leadership based upon the needs of the current situation. The following are several leadership approaches:

- Behavioral approach: the leader is considerate and supportive of team members; the leader provides directive to team members and specific tasks for completion; the leader demonstrates desired behaviors to team
- Relational approach: dyadic relationship between leaders and followers; leaders shape team members' perceptions of the environment
- Transformational approach: leader induces followers to transcend their interests for a greater good; characteristically involves inspiration and motivation
- Transactional approach: aimed at negotiating mutually beneficial exchanges with followers
- Contextual approach: recognition of the need to use a combination of approaches to meet situational requirements; may involve rotating leadership depending upon situation; may be the most effective for a physician leader of an organization or small clinic team

Q 13.2: a. Team development of a shared mental model of goals and responsibilities

Team effectiveness, also referred to as team performance, is a team's capacity to achieve its goals and objectives. This capacity to achieve goals and objectives leads to improved outcomes for the team members (e.g., team member satisfaction and willingness to remain together) as well as outcomes produced or influenced by the team.

Team processes are the means by which team members marshal and coordinate their individual resources to meet the demands of the task. When a team's cognitive, motivational, and behavioral processes become aligned with task demands, the team is effective. Team processes can be broken down as follows:

- Cognitive team processes: shared understanding of "task requirements, procedures, and role responsibilities" and the distribution of unique knowledge across team members
- Affective team processes: team cohesion, efficacy, and conflict have well-established relations with team effectiveness
- Behavioral team processes: individuals' knowledge and skills relevant to working in teams (i.e., competencies of working in a team) and team self-regulation/motivation affect how team members allocate their resources to perform tasks and adapt as necessary to accomplish goals

Suggested further reading

1. Cooke NJ, Hilton ML, eds. *Enhancing the Effectiveness of Team Science*. Washington, DC: National Academies Press; 2015.

Case 14 answers

Q 14.1: d. Long-term psychologic outcomes

Family members are considered a critical aspect of any patient care team, especially in the ICU. Both the manner in which communication between the health care team and family members occurs and the extent to which family is involved in decision making are known to affect long-term psychologic outcomes such as anxiety, depression, and posttraumatic stress disorder. Other studies have shown that family involvement in daily delirium reduction interventions, nutritional documentation, and promotion of mobility are acceptable and feasible to both ICU personnel and family members, but no long-term outcomes have been shown.

Suggested further reading

1. Donovan AL, Aldrich JM, Gross AK, et al. Interprofessional care and teamwork in the ICU. *Crit Care Med.* 2018;46:980-990.

Case 15 answers

Q 15.1: d. Synchronize interprofessional staffing and work scheduling

The implementation of the ABCDEF bundle (awakening and breathing coordination, delirium, early exercise/mobility, and family empowerment) has shown significant improvement in patient outcomes. One study including ICU patients in seven California hospitals revealed that for every 10% increase in total bundle compliance, odds of hospital survival increased by 15%. Bundle compliance also resulted in increased delirium-free and coma-free days. Barriers to implementation of this bundle are plentiful and related to the patient (e.g., patient instability, lack of cooperation), clinician (e.g., reluctance to follow protocol), the protocol itself (e.g., lack of clarity about who is responsible, lack of confidence in screening tools) or are related to the specific context of the ICU and those who work inside of it (e.g., lack of interprofessional care team coordination or staffing, staff turnover). Overcoming barriers first requires diagnosing the underlying etiology and then making concerted efforts to overcome identified barriers. One of the most difficult barriers to overcome is the coordination, communication, and collaboration among interprofessional care team members because of the many individuals involved in a patient's care and other competing demands for each of those team members that preclude collaboration. Hospitals and health systems consistently look for opportunities to increase care coordination without reducing efficiency or productivity of the care team members.

Suggested further reading

1. Costa DK. White MR. Ginier E. Manojlovich M. Govindan S. Iwashyna TJ. Sales AE. Identifying barriers to delivering the awakening and breathing coordination, delirium, and early exercise/mobility bundle to minimize adverse outcomes for mechanically ventilated patients: A systemic review. *Chest.* 2017;152(2):304-311.

10

Leadership in Health Care

Jennifer E. Schwartz, MD, FRCPC

Cases and questions

Case 1

Q 1.1: How do national organizations emphasize the importance of leadership?

a. They incorporate competencies into expectations for graduating trainees

b. They incorporate them into their models of expected behaviors

c. They create programs for physicians to improve their skill sets

d. All of the above

Case 2

Q 2.1: The rationale for clinician leadership includes which of the following?

a. Health care providers possess innate leadership skills

b. Physicians frequently resist change and therefore need adequate clinician leadership skills to address their resistance

c. There is evidence of improved patient outcomes when utilized

d. Physicians are often financially skilled, providing better fiscal oversight than nonclinician leaders

Case 3

Q 3.1: According to the Institute for Healthcare Improvement (IHI) Leadership Alliance, the four mental models for health care leaders include individuals and their families as partners in care, service alignment with payment systems, a focus on value, and what other model?

a. Person centeredness

b. Empowerment of all participants as improvers

c. Catalyzing change in health care

d. Authenticity in facilitating change

Case 4

A nurse notes an increased number of unexpected falls on his unit. He reviews the data and engages the floor manager who observes that all patients had negative fluid balances in the 3 days prior. He subsequently involves the patient safety director and, with his support, designs a pilot program of obtaining orthostatic blood pressures on patients with reduced oral intake. In the subsequent 3 months, the number of falls is reduced by 80%. The vice president of nursing is engaged, and policy is ultimately changed.

Q 4.1: What is this scenario an example of?

a. Front-line leadership

b. Executive leadership

c. Academic leadership

d. Team leadership

Case 5

Q 5.1: To develop health care leaders, common opportunities include which of the following?

a. Coaching and fellowships

b. Executive classes

c. Initiatives to address gaps in leadership

d. All of the above

Case 6

Q 6.1: Physicians are underrepresented in hospital leadership positions. In what way can other industries provide evidence to support their broader inclusion?

a. Executive leaders in other industries often have an in-depth understanding of the business they serve

b. Executives in other industries possess innate leadership skills

c. Executives in other industries often have a business background
d. Executives in other industries possess strong marketing skills

Case 7

The chief executive officer (CEO) of a health care system is selected to discuss leadership at her institution. She is asked to note the most important elements of leadership.

Q 7.1: Reflecting upon multiple models, she notes that, according to physician beliefs and physician leaders, the key competencies include all the following EXCEPT:
a. Interpersonal skills and communication
b. Professional ethics and responsibility
c. Emotional intelligence and vision
d. Financial and strategic planning

Case 8

Q 8.1: Interprofessional educational leadership models incorporate similar characteristics to the physician leader model. The Healthcare Leadership Alliance Model defines three domains. If a leader is said to possess expertise in analytical and innovative thinking, what would denote his or her domain of excellence?
a. Managing services
b. Execution
c. Transformation
d. People

Case 9

A health care leader tasks his team with reducing patient infection rates by 20% over the coming year. All departments and staff are asked to define how they will assist in meeting this goal by analyzing their processes and team needs, accordingly.

Q 9.1: This approach is consistent with which of the following?
a. Patient centeredness
b. Functional results–oriented health care leadership model
c. Toyota production system model
d. All of the above

Case 10

Q 10.1: To differentiate between trait theory and behavioral theory of leadership, trait theory implies which of the following?
a. Leadership can be taught
b. Leadership is innate
c. Leaders are defined by actions
d. Leaders are defined by interactions with others

Case 11

The department chair of medicine asks all division chiefs to determine a divisional fiscal policy that will permit the ongoing funding of medical educators. The department chair explains why this is critical to enhance her ability to attract the best educators and create outstanding learning opportunities for undergraduate and graduate learners within their individual divisions and the department as a whole, ultimately leading to increased retention and workforce expansion.

Q 11.1: This is an example of what type of leadership theory?
a. Transformational theory
b. Situational theory
c. Servant theory
d. Behavioral theory

Case 12

A clinician leader seeks to improve access to care for his patients in a grossly underserved area. Working tirelessly, he coordinates with multiple parties and facilitates a broader access program. When asked about his motivation, he replies, "It's all about my patients and improving their care."

Q 12.1: This is an example of what leadership theory?
a. Transformational theory
b. Situational theory
c. Servant theory
d. Behavioral theory

Case 13

Q 13.1: Maintaining patient centeredness and professionalism pertain to which competency category?
a. Self-management
b. Influence and communication
c. Systems-based practice
d. Health care foundations

Case 14

In the pursuit of excellence, leaders should create a culture in which goal achievement can be rewarded, where it is possible to clear barriers to success, the noble nature of the stated goal is ensured, others are motivated through empathy, and a clear, mutual understanding of team needs is developed.

Q 14.1: This pertains to which leadership competency domain?
a. Team management
b. Self-management
c. Influence and communication
d. Executing toward a vision

Case 15

A leader notes general discontent within a department. She provides the opportunity for all stakeholders to voice concerns and share their ideas. Thereafter, she carefully reads the annual reviews and personnel feedback about their leaders and the organization. In addition to considering her own behaviors, it becomes apparent that middle management has been unable to lead as effectively as possible. She decides to provide the managers with additional leadership training.

Six months later, outcomes and morale are markedly improved.

Q 15.1: This leader excelled in which competency domain?
a. Systems-based practice/management
b. Self-management
c. Team management
d. Health care foundations

Case 16

Q 16.1: What does the term *affirmative listening* refer to?
a. Active listening and engaging in conversation
b. Listening attentively and being open to suggestions
c. Listening effectively and ensuring comprehension of the topic
d. Listening with sincerity with the intent to learn and then act

Case 17

Politics and leadership are intertwined. When leaders create a vision, they must communicate effectively with all stakeholders, advocate for change inside and outside the organization, and take steps to understand the perspectives of those who support the vision as well as those who do not.

Q 17.1: The ability to have difficult conversations while continuing to communicate, negotiate, plan strategically, and build a team all reside in which competency domain?
a. Influence and communication
b. Team management
c. Systems-based practice
d. Health care foundations

Case 18

Q 18.1: To acquire the necessary skills to effect change within an ever-shifting landscape of health care, what avenues are available to leaders to increase their knowledge base?
a. Masters of Public Health
b. Masters in Health Care Administration
c. National organizations
d. All of the above

Case 19

A new leader is hired for a health care institution. He begins by analyzing the current financial data as well as the overall vision statement for the organization. In reviewing the current health care climate and needs assessment, he concludes that, while one of their programs has been very meaningful to the organization, it no longer makes fiscal sense to continue due to reduced funding opportunities and a reduced need within the greater community.

Q 19.1: This leader demonstrates which competency within systems-based practice/management?
a. Advocacy
b. Business knowledge and skills
c. Serving selflessly
d. Creating culture

Case 20

Q 20.1: To effectively create a culture of change, leaders must think creatively and consider new ideas to achieve success. If a leader wants to pilot a new approach, in addition to contextualizing it within a patient-centered framework and securing resources, what must a leader do?
a. Remain accountable
b. Concurrently apply a tried-and-true approach
c. Ensure that there is an expected 95% success rate
d. Ensure that standardized operating procedures are utilized

Case 21

Q 21.1: To successfully impact health care delivery, various business functions are required with associated training. To communicate effectively with the community at large and create a larger web-based presence, a leader may want to consider training in which area to be most effective?
a. Human resources
b. Marketing
c. Lean training
d. Accounting and finance

Case 22

Q 22.1: A CEO seeks to become a better leader to help execute her vision. She should pursue what further training?
a. Marketing
b. Accounting
c. An advanced degree
d. Human resources

Case 23

Q 23.1: What is a common launching pad for physician leaders in a formal setting?
a. Chief medical officer
b. Board of directors
c. Chief operations officer
d. Both a and b

Case 24

Q 24.1: Physician leadership often appears accidentally. What is the likely reason for this?
a. The physician's innate abilities to lead
b. The physician's commitment to patient care and health outcomes
c. The physician's understanding of operations and quality outcomes
d. Both b and c

Case 25

Q 25.1: What opportunities exist for physicians to apply leadership competencies outside of a formal role?
a. Guiding operational management
b. Advocating public policy
c. Impacting patient safety within their clinical environment
d. All of the above

Answers

Case 1 answers

Q 1.1: d. All of the above
There is a critical need for effective leadership within the health care field. To create health care transformation, physician leaders need to be trained to enhance team performance and to function effectively within an interprofessional environment. Organizations demonstrate their commitment to this endeavor by defining competencies for graduate trainees, defining new models of the physician role, and offering leadership learning opportunities at the national level.

Case 2 answers

Q 2.1: c. There is evidence of improved patient outcomes when utilized
While it is frequently assumed that physicians will resist change, this is not always the case. As has been supported in some of the literature, physicians are not always innate leaders, nor necessarily fiscally knowledgeable. However, evidence has shown that clinician leadership can improve patient outcomes, decrease expenditures, and improve efficacy and staff satisfaction.

Case 3 answers

Q 3.1: b. Empowerment of all participants as improvers
The IHI Leadership Alliance outlines the four mental models, including the three listed and the empowerment of all participants as improvers. These models provide a framework to achieve the Triple Aim, which includes improving the experience of care, improving the health of populations, and reducing the per capita costs of health care.

Case 4 answers

Q 4.1: a. Front-line leadership
Individuals on the front lines of patient care can exert situational leadership and can affect change. The ability to engage key stakeholders and communicate effectively can cause cultural changes and ultimately improve patient care.

Case 5 answers

Q 5.1: d. All of the above
The National Center for Healthcare Leadership focuses on the development of leaders. While pathways to leadership may vary, there remain various opportunities for people to obtain the skill set needed and to fill perceived gaps in their abilities.

Case 6 answers

Q 6.1: a. Executive leaders in other industries often have an in-depth understanding of the business they serve
Executives in other industries often possess an in-depth knowledge of the core business. This understanding can allow them to be more effective in addressing core values, implementing strategy, and communicating with stakeholders on the front lines. While they often do possess greater business acumen as well as a higher level of business functioning, these other selections do not support the inclusion of physicians as leaders who often do not possess that knowledge.

Case 7 answers

Q 7.1: d. Financial and strategic planning
Multiple models focus on competencies, including the ability to communicate effectively, to act in a professional and ethical manner, to possess emotional intelligence, and to have vision and initiative to impact the organization. Financial planning, while an aspect of the systems-based practice competency, does not represent a key competency according to physician leaders.

Case 8 answers

Q 8.1: c. Transformation
This model is governed by three domains: transformation, people, and execution. The people domain centers around the human elements of leadership, including relationship building, professionalism, and team leadership. Execution refers mainly to accountability, impact, influence, and process management, among other concepts. Transformation involves information seeking, analytical thinking, strategic orientation, and other elements. Managing services is not a domain in this model.

Case 9 answers

Q 9.1: d. All of the above
It is important to recognize that there is tremendous overlap in these models and aspects of leadership. Fundamentally, these models rely on the achievement of a unifying goal and the processes to render that possible. Whether in health care or in business, similar principles apply.

Case 10 answers

Q 10.1: b. Leadership is innate
Trait theory, such as the Great Man theory, implies that leadership is innate and predetermined. Behavioral theories state leadership is defined by interactions with others and one's actions, implying that leadership behaviors can be learned.

Case 11 answers

Q 11.1: a. Transformational theory
Transformational theory implies that leaders can motivate others by appealing to their idealism. The four *Is* are capitalized upon and include idealized influence, inspirational motivation, intellectual stimulation, and individualized consideration. The other theories listed utilize alternative approaches.

Case 12 answers

Q 12.1: c. Servant theory
Servant leadership argues that leaders influence followers by serving the needs of others. Situational theory implies that leadership effectiveness is affected not only by environmental factors but also by the characteristics of the subordinates and the nature of the work to be done. Transformational theory involves appealing to individuals' idealism rather than the population served.

Case 13 answers

Q 13.1: d. Health care foundations
The health care competencies encompass observed and measurable skills, knowledge, abilities, and personal attributes that leaders will demonstrate. They are divided into domains or categories, each of which include specific competencies. Leaders who make decisions that maintain a patient-centered focus and adhere to ethical professional standards demonstrate competence within the health care foundations category.

Case 14 answers

Q 14.1: b. Self-management
Health care competencies encompass observed and measurable skills, knowledge, abilities, and personal attributes that leaders will demonstrate. They are divided into domains or categories, each of which include specific competencies. The descriptors provided correspond to the competencies of serving selflessly, achievement orientation, pursuing excellence, and emotional intelligence which are listed within the self-management competency domain.

Case 15 answers

Q 15.1: c. Team management
Team management entails relationship management whereby leaders learn from criticism and improve from this information. Additionally, team management requires developing new talent. This leader clearly addresses those two elements. The other domains do not contain these competencies.

Case 16 answers

Q 16.1: d. Listening with sincerity with the intent to learn and then act
Affirmative listening is defined as listening with sincerity and the intent to learn and act. This aligns with a Just Culture in which subordinates feel comfortable voicing concerns without fear of repercussions or reprisal.

Case 17 answers

Q 17.1: a. Influence and communication
The ability to communicate effectively, advocate for your team and institution, have challenging conversations, and navigate politics are competencies within the influence and communication competency area. The other selections contain other competencies.

Case 18 answers

Q 18.1: d. All of the above
It is critical for leaders to master systems-based practice/management. One element within that area is knowledge of the health care environment. Effective leaders must be cognizant of evolving regulations, financial concerns, and the many health care models. Whether through obtaining additional degrees or by engaging with regional and national organizations, these all represent opportunities to gain further skill in this competency.

Case 19 answers

Q 19.1: b. Business knowledge and skills
This leader, while demonstrating knowledge of the health care environment, is utilizing business knowledge and skills to make data-driven decisions to help the organization as a whole. While the specific program has been historically meaningful, by analyzing the potential revenue and expense data, the leader can make effective planning decisions for the future, thus ensuring the organization remains solvent while maintaining its mission.

Case 20 answers

Q 20.1: a. Remain accountable
A leader must have a well-formed set of working relationships based on trust and accountability. Success often demands thinking outside the box, and a leader should endeavor to work around standard operating procedures and regulations to innovate, knowing full well that all ideas may not be successful.

Case 21 answers

Q 21.1: b. Marketing
When considering communications with the community at large through websites or enhanced community presence, leaders may want to pursue training in marketing to ensure that they are effective in their attempts to do so. The other answers provided, while appropriate in other circumstances, would not achieve the desired goal.

Case 22 answers

Q 22.1: c. An advanced degree
A CEO should pursue a more advanced degree that will likely encompass all of the other selections listed. The CEO must have strong executive functioning with knowledge about all aspects of the organization.

Case 23 answers

Q 23.1: d. Both a and b
Within health systems, elected or appointed positions (chief of staff, chief medical officer, or board of directors) usually serve as the initial foray into leadership. Physicians gain experience and exposure, permitting networking and broader understanding of multiple facets of the health system.

Case 24 answers

Q 24.1: d. Both b and c

Physician leaders are knowledgeable about a patient-centered vision, the day-to-day operations on the front lines, and the health care outcomes that need to be achieved. On that basis, physician leaders often find themselves in positions of leadership without formalized training. Because of the multiple competencies required for success, additional support and education is needed to supplement the inherent knowledge physicians possess.

Case 25 answers

Q 25.1: d. All of the above

While opportunities abound for formal leadership roles with requisite training and expertise, it is clear that physicians can be leaders in multiple settings in a health care organization outside of a formalized role. Whether it be through front-line leadership, impacting quality outcomes, guiding operational decisions from an informed perspective, or advocating for improved public health, physicians can demonstrate leadership competencies from any position.

Suggested further readings

1. Atchison TA, Bujak JS. *Leading Transformational Change: The Physician-Executive Partnership*. Chicago: Health Administration Press; 2001.
2. Barker A. *Improve Your Communication Skills*. London: Kogan Page; 2006.
3. Collins JC. *Good to Great and the Social Sectors: A Monograph to Accompany Good to Great*. Boulder, CO: Harper-Business; 2005.
4. Fisher R, Ury W, Patton B. *Getting to Yes: Negotiating Agreement Without Giving In*. New York: Penguin Books; 1991.
5. *HBR's 10 Must Reads on Leadership*. Boston: Harvard Business Review; 2011.
6. Quinn RE. Moments of greatness: entering the fundamental state of leadership. *Harv Bus Rev*. 2005;83(7): 74-83, 191.
7. Swensen S, Pugh M, McMullan C, Kabcenell A. *High-Impact Leadership: Improve Care, Improve the Health of Populations, and Reduce Costs*. Cambridge, MA: Institute for Healthcare Improvement; 2013.

11

Systems Thinking and Complexity Science

Maria Hamilton, MBA, Ami DeWaters, MD, MSc

Cases and questions

Case 1

Mr. K is discharged from the hospital and instructed to go to an appointment with his primary care physician (PCP) 3 days later, in compliance with the health care system's rule that all patients discharged from the hospital have a follow-up appointment within 7 days. He arrives at the outpatient appointment with his discharge instructions, which do not include an explanation for why he was in the hospital. His PCP does not have the same electronic health record (EHR) as the hospital, therefore the PCP has no record of what happened during his hospital stay. Mr. K tells his PCP that he was admitted for "problems with his insulin," and Mr. K was told by the discharging physician to discuss his insulin regimen with his PCP. The PCP decides to schedule another visit in a week once records from the hospitalization have been received, so that an informed decision can be made about how to adjust insulin for Mr. K. The patient leaves frustrated, feeling that his copay and time were wasted on an unnecessary visit.

Q 1.1: What aspects of the system drove the PCP's behavior and decision to schedule another visit so soon?
a. Communication at discharge
b. EHR interoperability
c. Patient's health literacy
d. Both a and b
e. All of the above

Q 1.2: What was the purpose that was driving this system's behavior?
a. Providing continuity of care
b. Reducing posthospitalization mortality
c. Reducing readmission rates
d. Shortening hospital length of stay

Q 1.3: What is one example of an element and an interconnection in the system outlined in the scenario?
a. Clinic, discharge instructions
b. Hospital, discharging physician
c. Hospital, EHR
d. None of the above

Case 2

The new chair of emergency medicine has decided that reducing the amount of time patients are in the emergency department is a top priority. To accomplish this goal, the emergency department staff wants to change the admission policy. Instead of calling other services and having to wait for them to come to admit patients, the emergency department staff wants their own physicians to place admission orders for each patient considered to be appropriate for admission, and the emergency department physician will decide to which service the patient should be admitted. Staff with the other departments in the hospital strongly disagree with the new policy and refuse to agree.

Q 2.1: What may be causing disagreement on this policy?
a. Some departments feel unintended consequences of the policy have not been considered
b. The departments have different mental models of admission criteria
c. Some departments disagree with the assumption that having their own physicians admit patients is lengthening the time patients are in the emergency department
d. Both a and c
e. All of the above

Q 2.2: A behavior-over-time graph would assist in addressing which of the concerns outlined in Question 2.1?
a. Unintended consequences
b. Differing mental models

c. The assumption that patients are lingering in the emergency department because of delays placing admission orders

d. None of the above

Case 3

A primary care clinic decides to implement an EHR for the first time. The first year after the EHR is put in place, the clinic receives approximately 1000 messages/month via the EHR. A year later, the number has increased to 10,000 messages/month. The clinic is suffering from high employee turnover, both among physicians and nursing staff, who are struggling to handle the influx of electronic messages. To address concerns, the clinic manager assesses all the messages coming into the clinic and divides them into categories (e.g., prescription refill requests, urgent concerns, requests for forms to be filled out). The manager then holds a meeting with all the staff to get agreement on which of the staff should be addressing which category of messages. After discussion, the staff agrees that physicians need to answer urgent concerns, the physician assistants will address prescription refill requests, and nurses can fill out most of the paperwork. The manager then hires a triage staff member to ensure the messages are sent to the appropriate person. After several months, the manager checks in to assess staff member burnout and finds the situation has improved for nurses and physicians, but the physician assistants are still being overwhelmed by prescription refill requests. The manager reviews the data and finds that renewing controlled substances is taking the most time and causing the most frustration; therefore refills for controlled substances are sent directly to the patient's primary care provider.

Q 3.1: How does this clinic demonstrate a complex adaptive system?

a. The clinic chooses not to reassess or iterate its messaging process

b. The clinic manager employs hierarchy to make decisions unilaterally

c. The clinic adapts multiple times to an increase in work that previously did not exist

d. None of the above

Q 3.2: How did the clinic manager first engage staff in the discussion of how to address messages?

a. The manager had a meeting to address mental models about which group should address which message

b. The manager gathered data on the types and number of messages that the clinic was receiving

c. The manager came in with a plan for how to address the messages and communicated that to the staff

d. Both a and b

e. All of the above

Q 3.3: Which of the following reinforcing and balancing loops best represents the clinic system?

a. (Fig. 11.1)

b. (Fig. 11.2)

c. (Fig. 11.3)

d. None of the above

Case 4

Q 4.1: Systems thinking links a person's environment to what characteristic?

a. Skills

b. Knowledge

c. Behavior

d. All of the above

Case 5

Q 5.1: What is the most important determinant of a system's behavior?

a. Function/purpose

b. Interconnections

c. Elements

d. Events

e. All of the above

Case 6

Q 6.1: Which of the following is a tool for surfacing and testing assumptions?

a. Ladder of inference

b. Stock and flow maps

c. Iceberg model

d. Behavior-over-time graphs

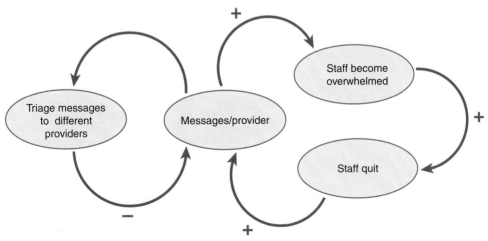

Fig. 11.1 Reinforcing and balancing loop option A.

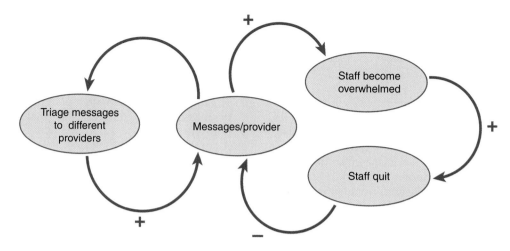

Fig. 11.2 Reinforcing and balancing loop option B.

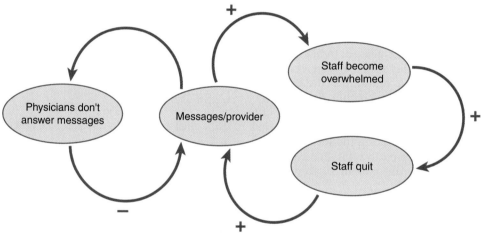

Fig. 11.3 Reinforcing and balancing loop option C.

Case 7

Q 7.1: Which of the following is NOT a habit of a systems thinker?
a. Mental models influence actions
b. Makes meaningful connections
c. Changes perspective to increase understanding
d. Understands every process can be broken down into its parts
e. Actions have consequences at multiple levels

Case 8

Q 8.1: What constitutes a system?
a. Relationships, feedback loops, reflections
b. Parts, connections, boundaries
c. Tools, methods, approaches
d. Interrelationships, perspectives, boundaries

Case 9

Q 9.1: How can complex adaptive systems be described?
a. Dynamic
b. Self-organized
c. Linear
d. Interdependent
e. Both a and c
f. Choices a, b, and d

Case 10

Q 10.1: Which of the following is an emerging property of a complex system?
a. Nested systems
b. Iteration
c. Self-organization
d. Instability
e. Simple rules
f. All of the above

Case 11

Q 11.1: What is the model used to explain systems thinking?
a. Design thinking
b. PDCA
c. Iceberg
d. Open systems theory

Case 12

Q 12.1: What is the correct order of levels within the iceberg framework?
a. Patterns, structures, events, mental models
b. Events, patterns, structures, mental models
c. Mental models, patterns, structures, events
d. Structures, mental models, events, patterns

Case 13

Q 13.1: What tools would be most effective in solving a problem at the patterns level of the iceberg model?
a. Causal loop
b. Behavior-over-time graph
c. Connection circles
d. Computer models
e. Ladder of inference

Case 14

Q 14.1: Complex adaptive systems are best described as systems that:
a. Can be understood by cause and effect in the system
b. Traditionally remain in equilibrium
c. Learn and adapt to changing environments
d. Build upon hierarchical relationships and rules

Case 15

Q 15.1: Which of the following is NOT an organizational system characteristic of a complex adaptive system?
a. Unpredictable
b. Adaptable
c. Controlling
d. Creative

Case 16

Q 16.1: Systems engineering is a branch of engineering concerned with:
a. Designing and managing complex systems
b. Designing physical and naturally built environments
c. Designing computer systems and integrating them into the larger picture
d. Both a and c
e. None of the above

Case 17

Q 17.1: What systems thinking tool would be most useful to computer modeling?
a. Habits of a systems thinker
b. Iceberg model
c. Connection circles
d. Stock and flow diagram

Case 18

Q 18.1: What systems thinking tool is used to illustrate reinforcing and balancing loops?
a. Behavior-over-time graphs
b. Connection circles
c. System archetypes
d. Causal loop diagrams

Answers

Case 1 answers

Q 1.1: e. All of the above
This case exemplifies how the system structure drives behavior. The primary care physician's (PCP) decision to delay any management decisions until a repeat appointment in 1 week was driven by his lack of knowledge about what happened during Mr. K's hospital stay. Several system structural factors contributed to this lack of knowledge: the lack of clear communication at discharge between the discharging physician and the PCP, the inability of the two different electronic health records to communicate with one another, and the patient's own inability to relate what occurred during his hospital stay.

Q 1.2: c. Reducing readmission rates
A system's purpose sets the direction of the system itself. This system's behavior was set by the rule to ensure that all patients discharged from the hospital had a follow-up appointment within 7 days of discharge. Many health care systems have a rule like this in place to reduce readmission rates. While the goal of reducing readmission rates is laudable, without the proper support in the rest of the system, many follow-up appointments can be underutilized due to lack of communication about what occurred during the hospitalization. One can imagine that if the system's purpose were to provide continuity of care, while all the elements and interconnections are still the same, the behavior would be quite different. Perhaps the system would have more extensive discharge instructions or require the electronic health records to communicate with one another.

Q 1.3: a. Clinic, discharge instructions
Elements in this system are the clinic, hospital, electronic health record, and discharging physician. An interconnection between many of the elements in the system is the discharge instructions, which were meant to connect the discharge physician's plan and the patient's course in the hospital to the primary care physician in the clinic.

Case 2 answers

Q 2.1: e. All of the above
In this case, department chairs may be utilizing several habits of a systems thinker which may raise concern about the new admission policy. The systems thinker first considers whether unintended consequences have been investigated. Department chairs may be concerned

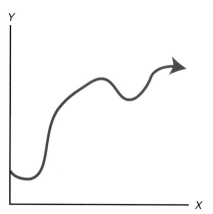

Fig. 11.4 Behavior-over-time graph. (Second Edition ©2014, 2010 Systems Thinking in Schools, Waters Foundation, www.watersfoundation.org.)

about how the workflow outside the emergency department will be affected by this new policy. Second, the systems thinker considers whether everyone in the system shares the same mental model. For example, there may be discordance between what emergency department physicians and other department physicians feel warrants an admission, exhibiting that different physicians working in the same system may not think similarly about the mental model for admission criteria for patients. Third, the systems thinker prefers not to make assumptions. Some of the department chairs may not be convinced that waiting for physicians outside the emergency department to place admission orders is what is causing patients to have long stays in the emergency department.

Q 2.2: c. The assumption that patients are lingering in the emergency department because of delays placing admission orders

In the iceberg model, assessing patterns of behavior with a behavior-over-time graph can be helpful in investigating the trends in the system. A behavior-over-time graph could be used to assess the amount of time it takes for physicians outside the emergency department to place admission orders, as well as the amount of time patients spend in the emergency department. This could help assess the assumption that the time patients spend in the emergency department is related to the time it takes for admission orders to be placed (Fig. 11.4).

Case 3 answers

Q 3.1: c. The clinic adapts multiple times to an increase in work that previously did not exist

A complex adaptive system is designed to be adaptable. The clinic in this case demonstrates adaptability several times: first by implementing an EHR, second by implementing a triage system, and third by changing the triage system when necessary. Complex adaptive systems are not hierarchical and persistently reassess system processes.

Q 3.2: d. Both a and b

The clinic manager in this case utilizes the iceberg model when considering change for the clinic system. The

manager starts by assessing patterns of behavior and gathers data on the types and numbers of messages being received. The manager then assesses the mental models of all the staff to determine if everyone agrees on who should be answering each type of message. As a manager of a complex adaptive system, she avoids taking a hierarchical approach and deciding for the staff how the messages will be handled.

Q 3.3: a. Fig. 11.1

Reinforcing and balancing loops are present in every system, and causal loop diagrams can help illustrate how the elements interact within a system. In this clinic, the messages/provider ratios are increasing, which in turn increases how overwhelmed the staff feel and leads to increased staff turnover. The loss of staff then leads to more messages/provider. This is the definition of a reinforcing loop. A balancing loop is put in place by triaging messages to different staff, reducing the messages/provider.

Case 4 answers

Q 4.1: c. Behavior

The central insight of systems theory is the relationship between structure and behavior. The overall structure of a system influences the individual's behavior working within that system (i.e., structure drives behavior). Since a system is a set of interconnected elements, it produces a certain behavior over time.

Case 5 answers

Q 5.1: a. Function/purpose

A system consists of three components: elements, interconnections, and a function/purpose. Elements are often the most recognizable piece of a system—the individual system parts. This could be the people working the clinic, the technology, the patients, and external providers. Interconnections represent the way the system is held together by relationships and how the various system elements work together. Function or purpose sets the direction of the system. A change in purpose dramatically changes a system, even if the elements and interconnections remain unchanged.

Case 6 answers

Q 6.1: a. Ladder of inference

The ladder of inference tool was developed by Chris Argyris to help practice the systems thinking habit of "surfaces and tests assumptions" (Fig. 11.5). This tool is primarily used to help in decision making from the point of receiving data to drawing conclusions. Stock and flow maps help with rates of change. The iceberg model is a framework for all elements of a system and challenges one to explore patterns, structural components, and mental models that may be influencing an identified behavior or event. Behavior-over-time graphs help with realizing goal achievement and demonstrates the behavior or performance of a system charted over time (see Fig. 11.5).

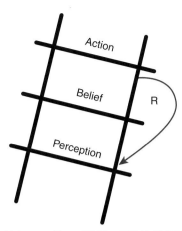

Fig. 11.5 Ladder of inference. (Second Edition ©2014, 2010 Systems Thinking in Schools, Waters Foundation, www.watersfoundation.org.)

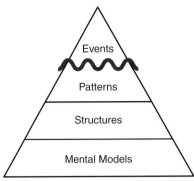

Fig. 11.6 The iceberg model. (Second Edition ©2014, 2010 Systems Thinking in Schools, Waters Foundation, www.watersfoundation.org.)

Case 7 answers

Q 7.1: d. Understands every process can be broken down into its parts
Reductionism is the theory that states you can understand every process by reducing it to its individual parts. Systems thinking is in contrast to reductionism and is concerned with how the parts interrelate and perform as a whole. The correct answer is choice d. All of the remaining answer choices are identified habits of a systems thinker.

Case 8 answers

Q 8.1: b. Parts, connections, boundaries
A system is a collection of parts that are connected for a common purpose. Systems both occur in nature and are also made by humans. All systems have boundaries that define the system and distinguish the system from other systems in the environment. For example, a freestanding urgent care center is a system that consists of various parts (i.e., people, technology, physical space). The boundaries of the urgent care center are defined by its scope, catchment area, and the characteristics of the patients it serves.

Case 9 answers

Q9.1: f. Choices a, b, and d
Of those listed there is only one choice that does not describe a complex adaptive system (CAS). By definition complex adaptive systems interact in nonlinear ways. CAS is an approach that challenges the standard problem-solving approach of cause and effect and sees the system as dynamic and dependent on relationships.

Case 10 answers

Q 10.1: f. All of the above
All of the answers to this question describe emerging properties of a complex adaptive system. Order cannot be predetermined in a CAS. Most systems are embedded within other systems (i.e., nested systems). One small change in the system can lead to significant system changes. The system follows simple rules and principles. Self-organization is a hallmark feature of a CAS as there is no center point of control or hierarchy.

Case 11 answers

Q 11.1: c. Iceberg
The iceberg model is the systems thinking tool that serves as a guide for looking at problems with a system's thinking lens (Fig. 11.6). It encourages exploration—not just looking at the event that happened but also at the patterns and trends over time, what structures were in place that influenced the event, and how mental models of the system participants are creating the system behavior. It allows for a more complete picture of different factors that may be contributing to system behavior (see Fig. 11.6).

Case 12 answers

Q 12.1: b. Events, patterns, structures, mental models
This is the primary model in systems thinking that helps observers to understand why things are happening the way they are. The observer of the system needs to recognize that whatever is going on in the system (what is "seen"; see Fig. 11.6) is rooted in the beliefs (mental models) of the participants in the system (what is "unseen"; see Fig. 11.6). If observers stop at the tip of the iceberg (events) then they can only react to the problem. If they can understand the patterns and the structures underneath the events and get to the mental models then they can begin to create the system transformation.

Case 13 answers

Q 13.1: b. Behavior-over-time graph
The behavior-over-time graph shows the relationship between time and the behavior of the system. It is the best choice of the tools listed to use at the patterns level within the iceberg model to begin to take individual events and determine if there are patterns to those events. It answers the question of why things are happening the way they are (see Fig. 11.4).

Case 14 answers

Q 14.1: c. Learn and adapt to changing environments
Complex adaptive systems have adaptation as a core feature of their design (e.g., human immune system, ant colonies, economy). Given some change within the environment those within the system are able to learn and therefore adapt their state.

Case 15 answers

Q 15.1: c. Controlling

Controlling is not a system characteristic of a complex adaptive system. A complex adaptive system refers to a system that emerges over time and adapts and organizes itself without a single point of control. There is no leader or individual who is coordinating the actions of others in the system.

Case 16 answers

Q 16.1: a. Designing and managing complex systems

The term *systems engineering* can be traced back to Bell Telephone Laboratories. It is a robust approach to design, creation, and operation of complex systems.

Case 17 answers

Q 17.1: d. Stock and flow diagram

System dynamics modeling packages use stocks and flows as their fundamental language making it much easier to build a computer model.

Case 18 answers

Q 18.1: d. Causal loop diagrams

All complex behavior is produced by either a reinforcing or a balancing loop. The causal loop diagram best demonstrates how the system either reinforces, balances, or negatively impacts the change.

Index